# A NEW HISTORY OF CATARACT SURGERY

# PART 6

# THE ERA OF SMALL-INCISION CATARACT SURGERY

edited by
Christopher T. Leffler

This is the standard softcover print-on-demand edition—an accessible and budget-friendly version of this work. For those who appreciate quality, a premium hardcover edition with high-quality color illustrations is also available. Visit our website for more information.

ISBN: 978-90-6299-481-6

Wayenborgh Publishing
P.O. Box 20538
1001 NM Amsterdam, The Netherlands
www.historyophthalmology.com



Wayenborgh Publishing is an imprint of Kugler Publications, P.O. 20538, 1001 NM, Amsterdam, The Netherlands

# Table of Contents

# 1. Evolution of Modern Cataract Surgery

Steven A. Newman, MD

In 1752, Jacques Daviel presented his technique for cataract extraction, as opposed to couching. Daviel used an extracapsular procedure with an opening in the anterior capsule, though some other surgeons used an intracapsular procedure in which the entire lens was removed. With the influence of Colonel Smith at the turn of the 20th century, intracapsular surgery became more popular (Smith 1926). Intracapsular extraction was sometimes aided by mechanically breaking the lens zonules (Jackson 1920) and forceps were designed to hold on to the lens (Verhoeff 1916). Beginning in the 1960s, the lens zonules could be enzymatically dissolved (Hill & Barraquer 1962) and the lens could be frozen with the cryoprobe (Fig. 1, Krwawicz 1961, Kelman 1967).

The use of intraocular lenses (IOLs), mentioned centuries ago, but successfully pioneered by Harold Ridley in the late 1940s, was groundbreaking (Ridley 1951, 1952). Ridley placed his IOL in the capsular bag, but several investigators suggested the use of anterior chamber lenses (Apple et al. 1987). At the time of Ridley's initial presentation in 1951, most cataract surgery was done using an intracapsular technique (entirely removing the lens in its capsule, sometimes aided by zonulolysis) (Ridley 1951). Many of the early IOLs used clips to the iris to hold them in place (Binkhorst 1973). No matter how the IOL surgery was performed, complications could still occur (Apple et al. 1987). For a significant time, there was a debate about the appropriate position for an IOL (in the bag, or in the ciliary sulcus in front of the anterior capsule). This has been generally decided in factor of placement in the capsular bag (Shearing 1981, Reidy et al. 1985). IOLs were Food and Drug Administration (FDA) approved and became commonly used, in the 1980s.

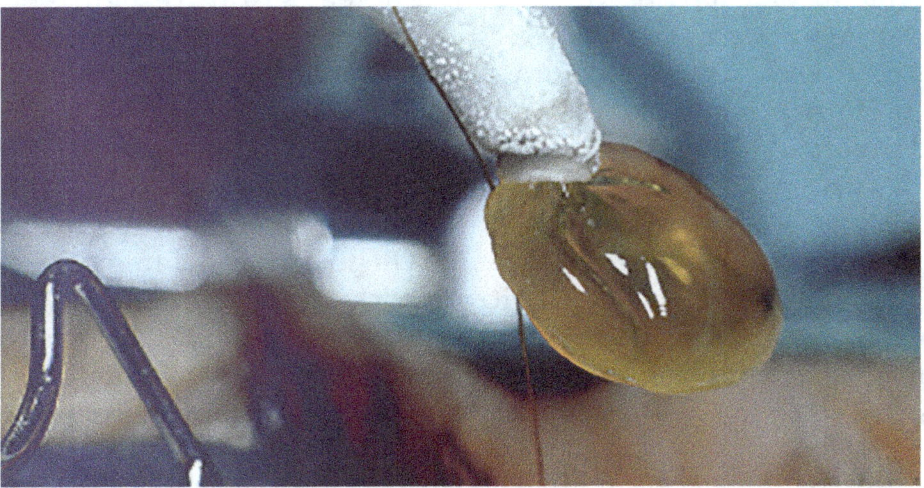

**Fig. 1.** Attachment of the cryoprobe to the crystalline lens.

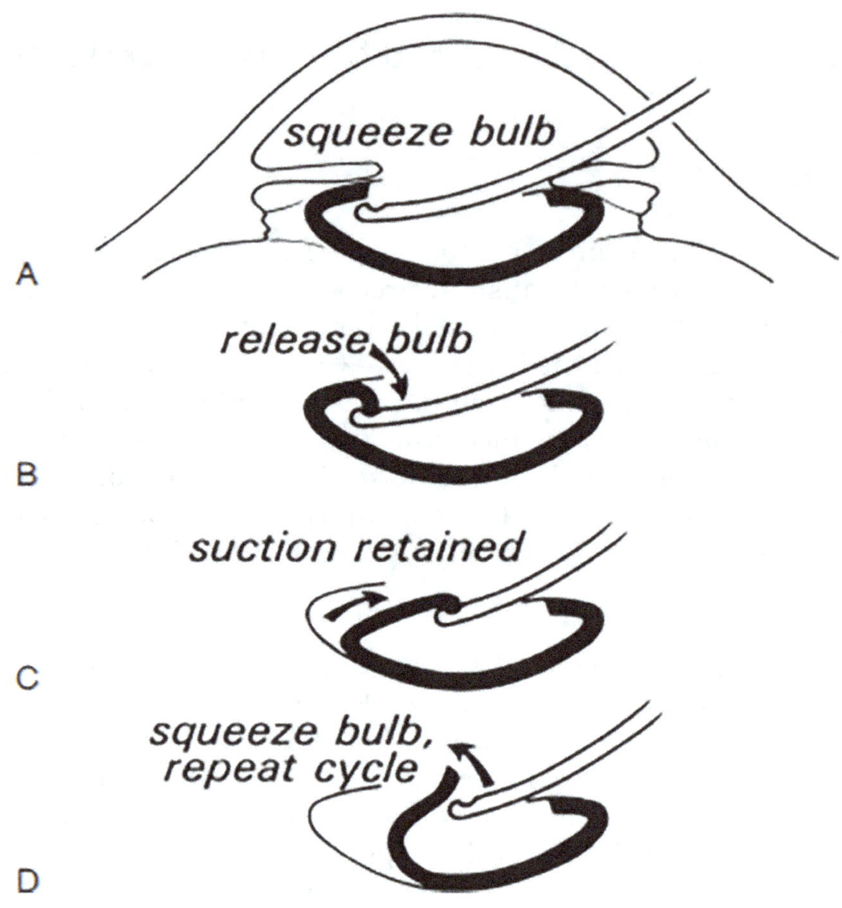


**Fig. 2.** "Microerisiphake" extraction of lens cortex by suction.

In 1967, Charlie Kelman ushered in a revolution in cataract surgery with his introduction of phacoemulsification (Kelman 1967, 1975). Kelman's desire was to make a small incision for cataract surgery, to reduce or eliminate the need for hospitalization postoperatively (Shepherd 1989). The development of phacoemulsification came after Charlie, working on a 3-year grant, recognized that lenses in young and pediatric patients were soft and could be aspirated (Fig. 2, Faust 1984), but adult lenses were hard and needed to be divided up before they could be removed. He had some interesting ideas about breaking up the nucleus, including putting it in a bag and crushing it.

One day Kelman was sitting in his dentist's office when he was shown a Cavitron, which dentists used to clean tartar off teeth. The first phacoemulsification machines were simply an adaptation of the Cavitron, with irrigation to keep the probe from getting too hot, plus aspiration to remove the lens fragments. Several modes were available, including burst mode to break up the lens (Baykara et al. 2006). Donald Gass suggested the use of a side-opening needle to help remove cortex (Gass 1969).

The evolutionary aspect of modern cataract surgery followed Kelman's introduction. Surgeons recognized that there were better ways of opening the anterior

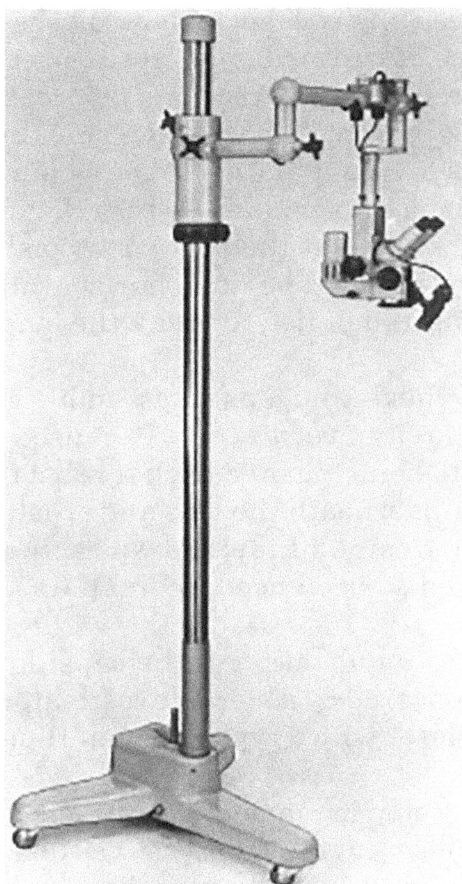

**Fig. 3.** Original Zeiss operating microscope.

capsule than the Christmas tree or multiple punctures. This was largely pioneered by Howard Gimbel, who spent time at the University of California in Irvine and subsequently returned to Canada (Gimbel & Neuhann 1990). A continuous tear capsulorrhexis could be created by tearing the anterior capsule. Dr. Gimbel used the Utrata forceps to make the puncture and start the incision, although one could certainly use a cystitome to open the capsule and either complete the incision and tear, or at least start it and prepare for the use of the Utrata (Gimbel 1991a).

Other changes included the use of magnification. Cataract surgeries were performed with loupes by a majority of surgeons through much of the 1960s (Keeler 2020). By the time I was a resident in the late 1970s, cataract surgeons used the operating microscope (Fig. 3).

A second major evolutionary aspect was the advent of separating the nucleus from the capsular bag. This could be done through hydrodissection and hydrodelineation, in which a cannula is placed just under the anterior capsule breaking the adhesions of the cortex to the capsule (Anis 1990, 1994; Fine 1992). Hydrodelineation could also be done where the cannula is placed between the cortex and the nucleus and an additional plane of separation was created.

Dr. Gimbel also introduced the concept of lens disassembly into smaller pieces, which decreased the chance of rupturing the posterior capsule and made removal of the lens fragments safer. This was first done by creating a groove and splitting the nucleus in half, essentially rotating and then splitting it into quarters (Gimbel 1991b, Gimbel & Debroff 2004). Japanese surgeons pioneered the idea of using a chopper to help break the lens into smaller pieces (Nagahara 1993). This was originally done with a Sinskey hook, but the pick was too sharp and could potentially damage the capsule. Chopping could be done horizontally, where the chopper was placed at the edge of the lens and pulled to break the lens along a line (Olson 2004).

Continuous tear capsulorrhexis and lens disassembly substantially decreased the risk of complications, although never to zero. Because I do not like the idea of an instrument, even if it is dull, being pushed back toward the posterior capsule, I will often place a Connor wand underneath the lens and crush the lens, separating it into pieces against the phaco tip. A similar method was actually suggested in the 1980s (Fig. 4). The YAG laser has also been used to break up the lens (Chambless 1988).

Another advance was the visualization of the capsule, especially with a mature white cataract. This was pioneered by several investigators, first with ICG green dye (Horiguchi et al. 1998) and later with Trypan (Vision Blue) dye (Sharma et al. 2002).

An additional evolutionary step in managing cataracts was anesthesia. When I was a resident in the late 1970s, most cataract surgery was done under general anesthesia. This was followed by the use of retrobulbar or peribulbar blocks (Atkinson 1936). The disadvantage of the retrobulbar block is that it has been associated with globe puncture and interference with motility (Golnik et al. 2000). Adaptations of local anesthesia have included peribulbar blocks and subtenon's injection with a blunt cannula (Stevens 1992). Even more recently, local anesthesia has been administered intraocularly (Gills et al. 1997). This can be done either alone or with conscious sedation.

Since Ridley first put a round lens without haptics in the eye (Ridley 1951), there has been a tremendous evolutionary advancement in IOLs. Initially, lenses were iris fixated (Fig. 5, Binkhorst 1973), but this could cause dislocation or inflammation (Apple et al. 1984). Other approaches included anterior chamber lenses supported in the angle (Binkhorst 1973, Reidy 1985) (Fig. 6) and, later, posterior chamber lenses that were given haptics that allowed them to center in the intact bag. Dr. Gimbel also pioneered the use of posterior optic capture in case of a tear in the posterior capsule (Gimbel 2001). This allowed the haptics of an IOL to be placed in the sulcus and yet be stabilized centrally with posterior capture (Gimbel & Amritanand 2013).

An additional evolutionary development was the use of viscoelastic. Viscoelastic first derived from rooster comb and had been used by Dr. Machemer for posterior segment surgeries as he felt that once the vitreous was removed, it had to be replaced. As it turns out, he discovered fairly rapidly that this step was unnecessary, as the vitreous was simply replaced by aqueous secreted by the ciliary body (Balazs et al. 1972).

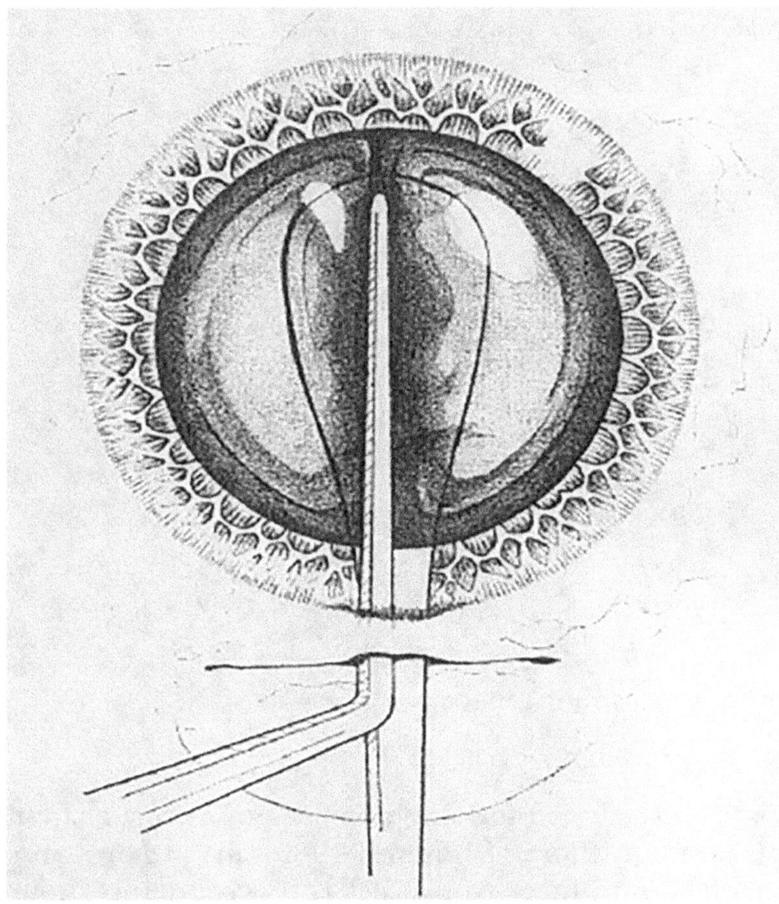

**Fig. 4.** Pressing both the nucleotome downward and the vectis upward, to bisect the nucleus, as performed by Peter Kansas by 1988.

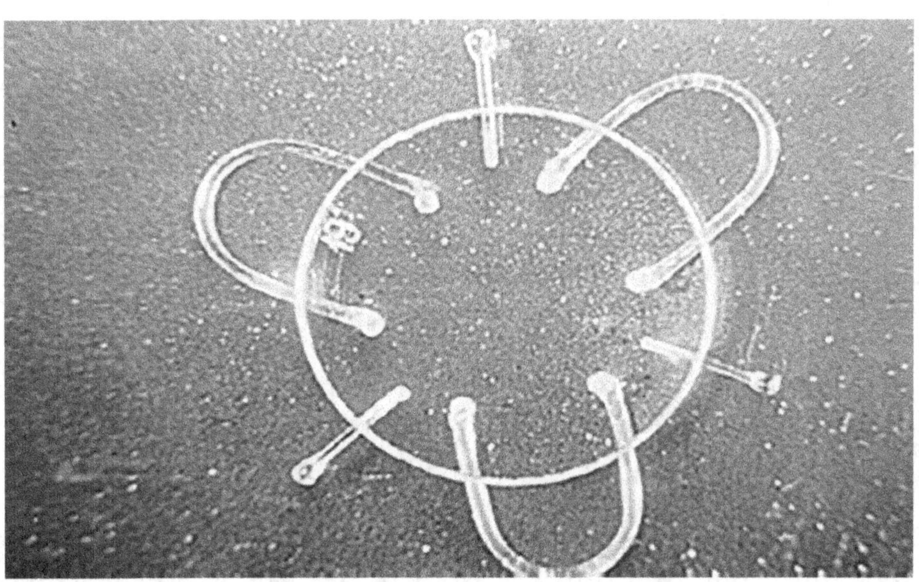

**Fig. 5.** The design of the Fyodorov-Zakharov iris-clip lens.

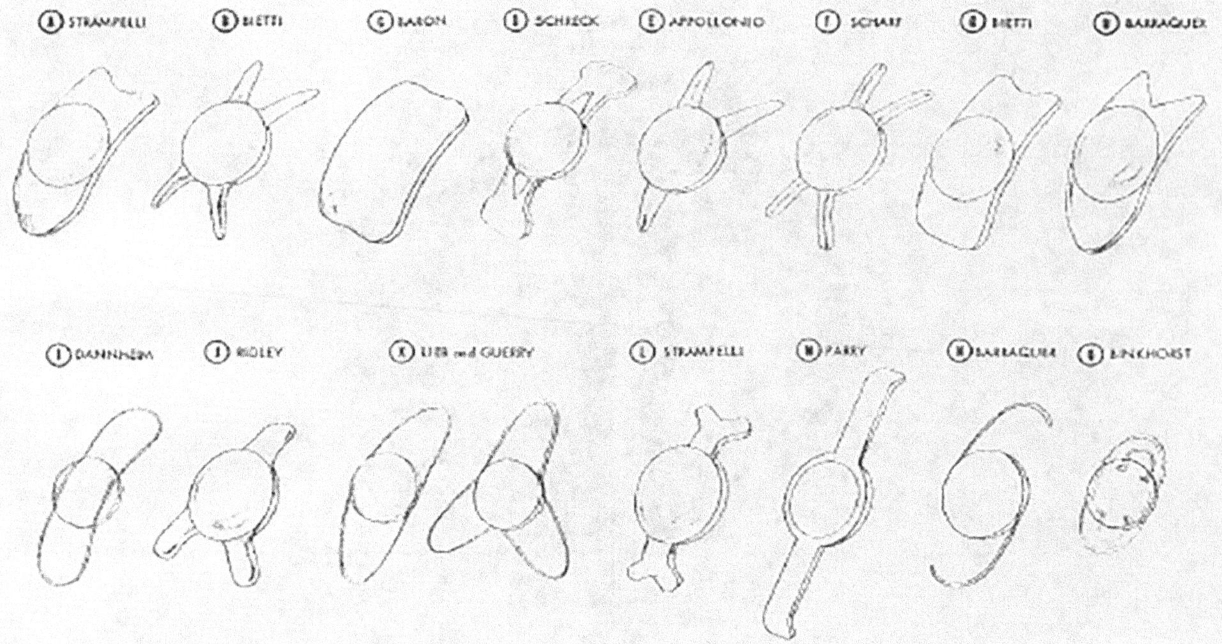

**Fig. 6.** Early anterior chamber lenses.

Viscoelastic was reintroduced for the purposes of anterior segment surgery by Dr. Miller at Beth Israel (Miller & Stemann 1980), first to protect the endothelium when inserting an IOL and later to protect the eye during the entire procedure (Liesegang 1984). The original viscoelastic patented in 1979, Healon, was made of hyaluronic acid and is cohesive and easier to remove, because it comes out in a single aspiration. The year 1985 saw approval of the first dispersive viscoelastic, Viscoat, which includes chondroitin sulfate as an ingredient and is able to coat the corneal endothelium and anything else you want to protect.

One additional advancement has been the shift of cataract surgery from an inpatient procedure. I remember making the rounds on patients who were admitted on Friday night for surgery the next morning. The advent of outpatient cataract surgery also drove the development of freestanding (ambulatory) surgery centers. Jimmy Gills, who trained in uveitis and neuro-ophthalmology, was really primarily responsible for introducing outpatient surgery in Spring Hills Florida. Gills founded the Saint Luke's Eye Clinic in 1968, and the practice became dedicated to IOL implantation in 1974, well ahead of other facilities in the United States (Gills 1975).

Another evolutionary invention was the development of foldable lenses. Lack of a foldable lens meant that we could do phacoemulsification through a 3 mm or less incision but then had to open the incision up to put the lens in. The first foldable lens, the Mazzocco Taco (Mazzocco et al. 1986), could be put through an incision less than 3 mm. Some of the original lens material was silicone. Unfortunately, this material could refold and find its way through the posterior capsule into the vitreous cavity (Petersen et al. 2000).

Following the taco lens, lenses were folded manually for insertion, and more recently, lenses have been placed into cartridges that allow them to be placed through a sub-3-mm incision, directing the haptics into the prepared bag. More recently, cartridges with preloaded lenses have been developed to make insertion easier.

The switch to clear corneal incision in the 1990s further reduced the opening into the eye and thus reduced the amount of induced astigmatism.

Additional methods of splitting the nucleus have included cross-action forceps that force the blades apart. This technique has not been particularly popular. More recently, femto lasers have been used to break up the lens before surgery. I am skeptical of the role that the femto laser will play in the future. The laser adds an extra expense and unfortunately does a fairly poor job of creating access incisions as well as performing the capsulorrhexis. I suspect that manual phacoemulsification cataract surgery will remain the standard of care, at least in developed countries, for the foreseeable future.

Although there will never be an operation that cannot cause complications, modern cataract surgery has become one of the safest surgical procedures.

# References


Anis AY. Refinements to the hydrodelineation technique. *Ocul Surg News*. 1990;8:32.

Anis AY. Understanding hydrodelination: the term and the procedure. *Doc Ophthalmol*. 1994;87:123-137.

Apple DJ, Mamalis N, Loftfield K, Googe JM, Novak LC, Kavka-Van Norman D, Brady SE, Olson RJ. Complications of intraocular lenses. A historical and histopathological review. *Surv ophthalmol*. 1984 Jul 1;29(1):1-54.

Apple DK. Hansen SP. Richards SC, Park RB, et al. Anterior chamber lenses. Part I. Complications and pathology and a review of designs. *J Cataract Refract Surg* 1987; 13:157-74.

Atkinson WS. Retrobulbar injection of anesthetic within the muscular cone. *Arch Ophthalmol*. 1936 Sep 1;16(3):494-503.

Balazs EA, Freeman MI, Kloti R, et al. Hyaluronic and aqueous humor. *Mod Probl Ophthalmol*. 1972;10:3-21.

Baykara M, Ercan I, Ozcetin H. Microincisional cataract surgery (MICS) with pulse and burst modes. *Eur J Ophthalmol* 2006;16:804-8.

Binkhorst CD. The iridocapsular (two-loop) lens and the iris clip (four loop) lens in pseudophakia. *Trans Am Acad Ophthalmol Otolaryngol*. 1973;77:589.

Chambless WS: Neodymium: YAG laser phacofracture: an aid to phacoemulsification. *J Cataract Refract Surg*. 1988;14:180-181.

Faust KJ. Hydrodissection of soft nuclei. *J Am Intraocul Implant Soc*. 1984;10:75-7.

Fine IH. Cortical cleaving hydrodissection. *J Cataract Refract Surg*. 1992;18:508-12.

Gass JD. Lens aspiration using a side-opening needle. *Arch Ophthalmol*. 1969 Jul 1;82(1):87-90.

Gills JP. Intraocular lens in perspective. *Eye Contact Lens*. 1975 Jul 1;1(3):39-48.

Gills JP, Cherchio M, Raanan M. Unpreserved lidocaine to control discomfort during cataract surgery using topical anesthesia. *J Cataract Refract Surg*. 1997;23:545-50.

Gimbel H, Neuhann T. Development advantages and methods of the continuous circular capsulorhexis technique. *J Cataract Refract Surg*. 1990;16:31-7.

Gimbel HV. Continuous curvillnear capsulorhexis and nuclear fracturing: evolution, technique, and complications. *Ophthalmol Clin North Am*. 1991a;4:235.

Gimbel HV. Divide and conquer nucleofractis phacoemulsification: development and variations. *J Cataract Refract Surg*. 1991b;17:281-91.

Gimbel HV, Sun R, Ferensowicz M, Penno EA, Kamal A. Intraoperative management of posterior capsule tears in phacoemulsification and intraocular lens implantation. *Ophthalmology*. 2001;108(12):2186-9.

Gimbel HV, Debroff BM. Intraocular lens optic capture. *J Cataract Refract Surg*. 2004; 30:200-6.

Gimbel HV, Amritanand A. Reverse optic capture to stabilize a toric intraocular lens. *Case Rep Ophthalmol*. 2013;4:138-43.

Golnik KC, West CE, Kaye E, et al. Incidence of ocular misalignment and diplopia after uneventful cataract surgery. *J Cataract Refract Surg*. 2000;26:1025-209.

Hill HF, Barraquer J. Some aspects of the use of enzymatic zonuloysis. *Am J Ophthalmol*. 1962;54:89-95.

Horiguchi M, Miyake K, Ohta I, Ito Y. Staining of the lens capsule for circular continuous capsulorrhexis in eyes with white cataract. *Arch Ophthalmol*. 1998 Apr 1;116(4):535-7.

Jackson E. Cataract operations. *Am J Ophthalmol*. 1920;3:774-6.

Keeler R. The history of the surgical microscope in ophthalmology. In: Leffler CT (ed.). *The History of Glaucoma*. Amsterdam: Wayenborgh, 2020; pp. 481-512.

Kelman CD. Phaco-emulsification and aspiration. A new technique of cataract removal. A preliminary report. *Am J Ophthalmol*. 1967;64:23-35.

Kelman CD. Phacoemulsification and aspiration: the Kelman technique of cataract removal. Birmingham, AL: Aesculpaius Pub Com, 1975.

Krwawicz T. Intracapsular extraction of intumescent cataract by application of low temperature. *Br J Ophthalmol*. 1961;45:279-86.

Liesegang TJ, Bourne WM, Ilstrup DM. Short and long-term endothelial cell loss associated with cataract extraction and intraocular lens implantation. *Am J Ophthalmol*. 1984;97:32.

Mazzocco TR, Rajacich GM, Epstein E, eds. *Soft implant lenses in cataract surgery*. New Jersey: Slack, 1986.

Miller D, Stemann R. Use of Na-hyaluronate in anterior segment eye surgery. *J Am Intraocul Implant Soc*. 1980;6:13-15.

Nagahara K. Phaco Chop Film presented at International Congress on Cataract. *IOL and Refractive Surgery*. Seattle: ASCRS, 1993 May.

Olson RJ. Clinical experience with 21-gauge manual microphacoemulsification using Sovereign WhiteStar Technology in eyes with dense cataract. *J Cataract Refract Surg*. 2004 Jan 1;30(1):168-72.

Petersen AM, Bluth LL, Campion M. Delayed posterior dislocation of silicone plate-haptic lenses after neodymium: YAG capsulotomy. *J Cataract Refract Surg*. 2000 Dec 1;26(12):1827-9.

Reidy JJ, Apple DJ, Goorge JM, et al. An analysis of semiflexible, closed-loop anterior chamber intraocular lenses. *Am Intraocular Implant Soc J*. 1985;11:344.

Ridley H. Intra-ocular acrylic lenses. *Trans Ophthalmol Soc UK*. 1951;71:617.

Ridley H. Intra-ocular acrylic lenses: a recent development in the surgery of cataract. *Br J. Ophthalmol*. 1952;36:113-12.

Sharma N, Gupta V, Vajpayee RB. Trypan-blue-assisted posterior capsule plaque removal. *J Cataract Refract Surg*. 2002 Jun 1;28(6):916-17.

Shearing SP. Evolution of the posterior chamber intraocular lens. *Am Intraocular Implant Soc J*. 1981;7:55.

Shepherd JR. Induced astigmatism in small incision cataract surgery. *J Cataract Refract Surg.* 1989;15:85-8.

Smith H. A new technique for the expression of the cataractous lens in its capsule. *Arch Ophthalmol.* 1926;55:213-24.

Stevens JD. A new local anesthesia technique for cataract extraction by one quadrant sub-Tenon's infiltration. *Br J Ophthalmol.* 1992;76:670-4.

Verhoeff FH. Improved capsule forceps for intracapsular cataract extractions. *Tr Am Ophth Soc.* 1916;12:489-94.

# 2. Charles Kelman and the Development of Small Incision Cataract Surgery (1965)

Christopher T. Leffler, MD, MPH[1]

## Introduction

Charles Kelman (1930-2004) developed small incision cataract surgery in the 1960s, by modifying a dental tool, the Cavitron ultrasonic instrument, to emulsify cataracts before they are removed from the eye (Fig. 1). Kelman was called Charlie by his friends and colleagues.

We reviewed the 400-page file of the John A. Hartford Foundation, which funded Kelman's research. We also conducted interviews between September and December 2023 with several people who knew Kelman, including his first wife, Joan Bernstein, who has never previously spoken to any historians. We interviewed Kerry Kuhn, MD, whose father, Larry Kuhn, DDS, was Kelman's dentist. Father and son Kuhn had discussed the involvement of Larry Kuhn in the development of phacoemulsification. Two sources, a 1972 profile and a 2010 documentary, included

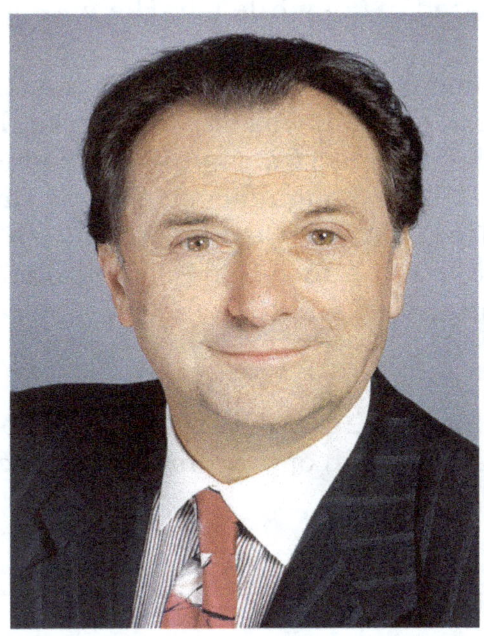

**Fig. 1.** Ophthalmologist Charles Kelman of New York (1930-2004).

---

1  Department of Ophthalmology. Virginia Commonwealth University. Richmond, VA, and the Department of Ophthalmology. Hunter Holmes McGuire VA Medical Center, Richmond, VA.

statements from both Kelman and Larry Kuhn.[2] We interviewed William Banko, the son of Cavitron engineer Anton Banko, who worked with Kelman to develop the first phacoemulsifier. Banko provided us with his father's lecture notes. We also interviewed two people who were working in Kelman's lab by 1965: Ronald B. Odrich, DDS, a dentist, and Cheryl Jalbert, *née* Chase, an assistant. We also interviewed Odrich's son, Marc Odrich, who is an ophthalmologist at the University of Virginia. At the Cogan Ophthalmic History Society meeting at Bascom Palmer, in Miami, April 19-21, 2024, we spoke with Norman Medow, who trained with Kelman first as a resident for 3 years, beginning in 1969, and then as a fellow. Medow also knew Ronald Odrich's sons, who were ophthalmologists. We interviewed Kelman's daughter, Lesley Koeppel.

# Education (1950–)

Kelman's father was an inventor. According to Joan, Kelman held his father in awe. Kelman used his father's name, David, as a middle name, even though that was not his actual middle name.[3] In 1966, Kelman thanked "David J. Kelman, my father, whose wisdom helped me to choose a medical career."[4]

Kelman graduated from Tufts University with a bachelor of science in 1950. At the University of Geneva in Switzerland, he earned a bachelor of medical science degree in 1952 to prepare him for medical school, followed by a medical degree in 1956.[5] Charlie's father passed away while Charlie was studying overseas.

On the ship returning home, Kelman befriended Sidney (Sid) N. Miller, an ophthalmologist from Poughkeepsie. Kelman was sitting in with the band on the cruise, and Miller asked if he could play Kelman's saxophone, a request that Kelman granted. Kelman ended up touring Miller's Poughkeepsie practice and becoming interested in ophthalmology. They continued to be friends.[6] In 1965, Kelman traveled to Poughkeepsie.[7] In 1966, Kelman listed himself as "Consultant Ophthalmologist, Vassar Brothers Hospital, Poughkeepsie," and thanked "Sidney N. Miller, MD, who imbued me with his love for ophthalmology."[8]

Kelman conducted his internship at Kings County Hospital from 1956 to 1957 and performed postgraduate work in ophthalmology at the Bellevue Medical Center

---

2 Vachon, 1972; Anker, 2010.

3 Personal communication with Joan Bernstein, Nov. 4, 2023.

4 Kelman, 1966, "Cryosurgical techniques," dedication page.

5 Kelman, Hartford Foundation Grant, Nov. 1963.

6 No author listed, *Ocular Surgery News*, 2002.

7 Hartford Foundation files, 1963-1972.

8 Kelman 1966, "Cryosurgical techniques," dedication page.

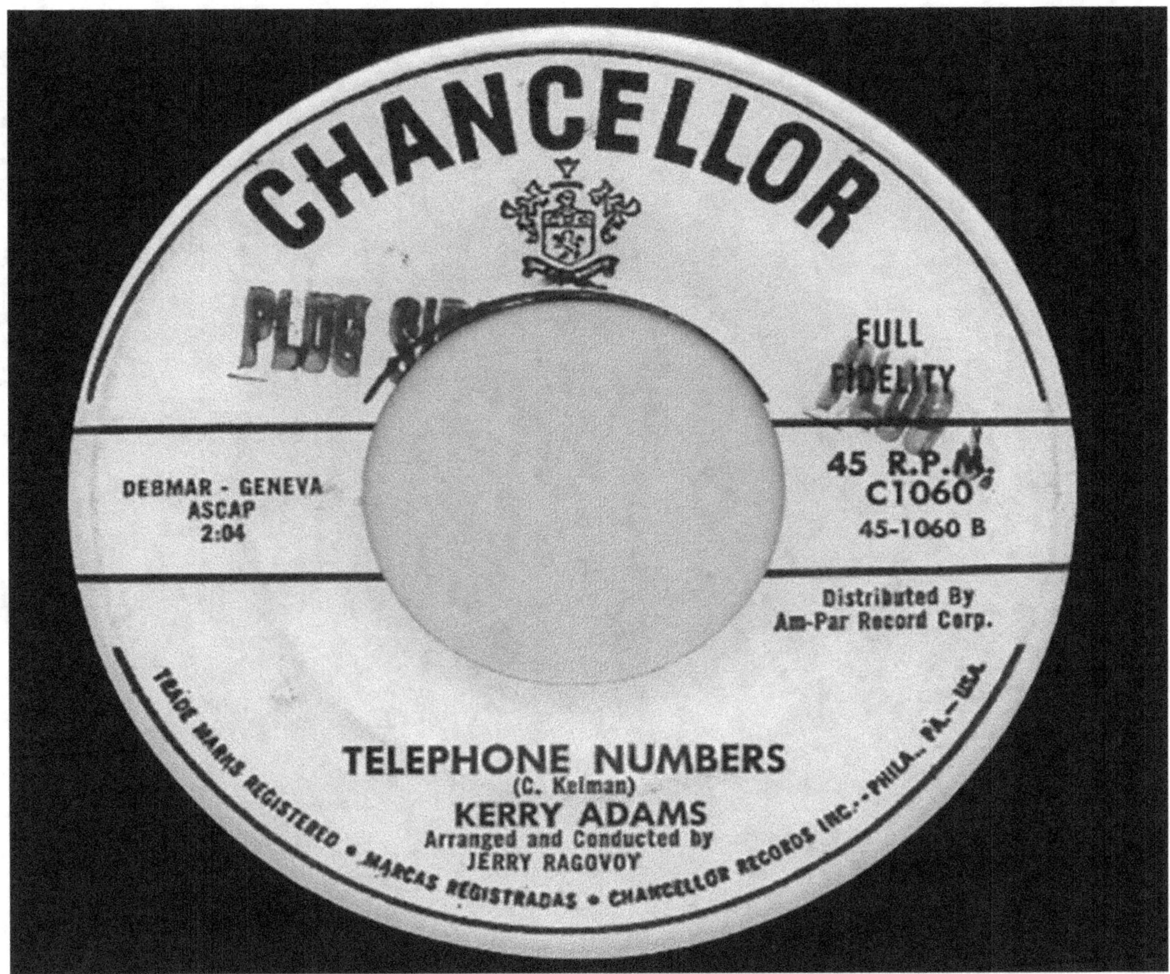


**Fig. 2.** The song *Telephone Numbers* by Kerry Adams (aka Charles Kelman) was on the Billboard Charts the week of October 10, 1960.

from 1957 to 1958, before completing his ophthalmology residency at Wills, in Philadelphia, from 1958 to 1960.[9]

On the Billboard Charts the week of October 10, 1960, Kelman had a hit under the pseudonym Kerry Adams called *Telephone Numbers*, about getting girls' phone numbers. He wrote the song and sang it himself (Fig. 2).

After his ophthalmology residency, Kelman practiced in New York, beginning in 1960. Kelman and his first wife Joan met at a restaurant in October 1961, when Charlie was 31 and Joan was 20 (Fig. 3).[10] Joan says that when they met, his doctor's bag was full of 45 records and he still hoped to make it big as a musician. They got engaged in December 1961. Joan was from Queens and had worked since she was in high school at age 17 years in 1958 in the dental office of Lawrence (Larry)

---

9 Kelman, Hartford Foundation grant, Nov. 1963.

10 Interviews with Joan Bernstein and Lesley Koeppel 2023.

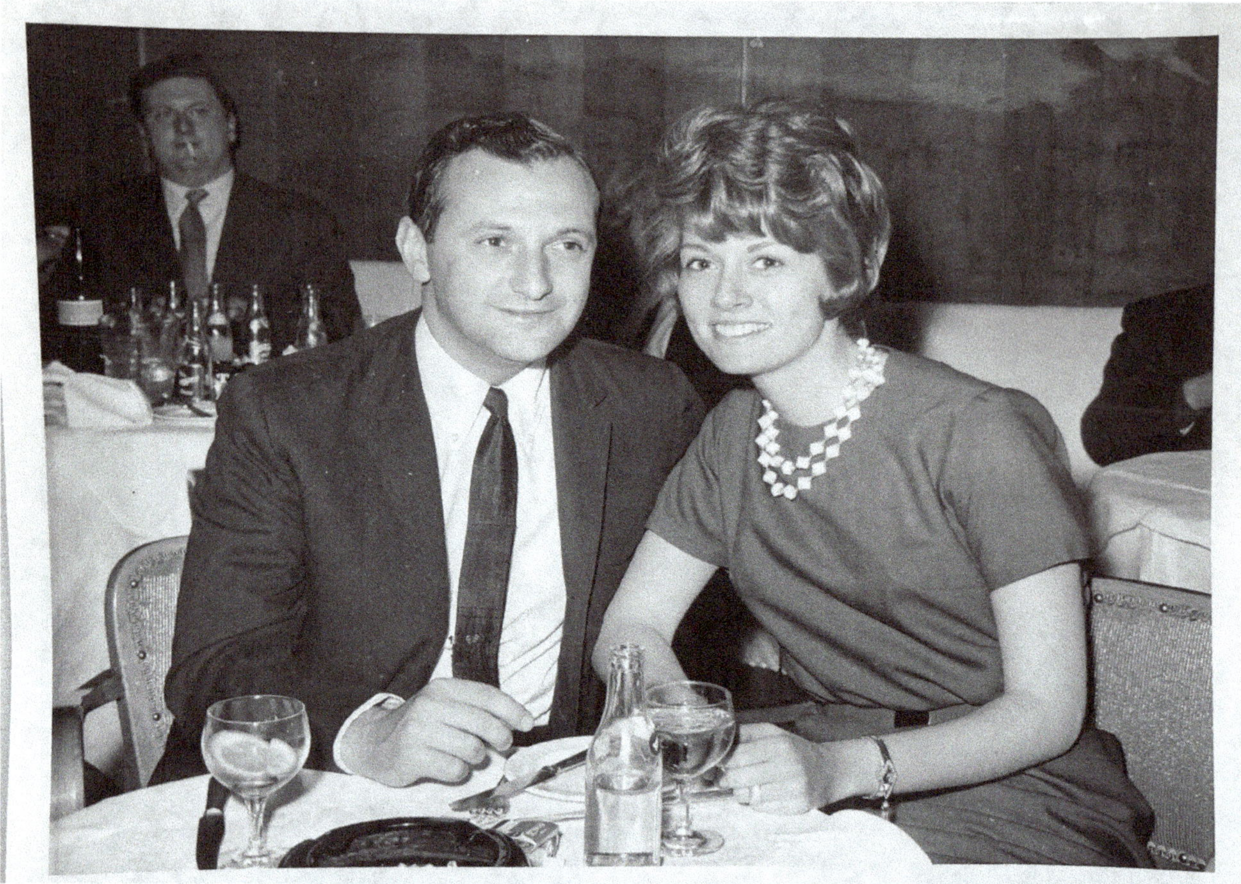

**Fig. 3.** Charles Kelman and his wife Joan on their honeymoon in April 1962.

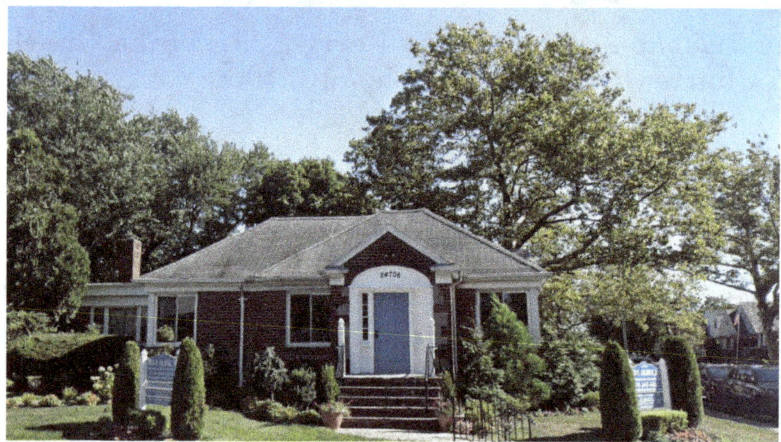

**Fig. 4.** Dental office of Lawrence (Larry) Kuhn at 247-06 Union Tpke, Bellerose, in Queens, New York, where Kelman's first wife Joan worked prior to their marriage. The office still houses a dental practice today.

Kuhn, whose office was at 247-06 Union Tpke, Bellerose (Fig. 4). Kuhn's office was also his home, and Joan could hear his wife Bunny dealing with the children sometimes. Kuhn's office was across the street from the home where Joan lived with her parents until she got married. Initially, she just helped with office tasks after school, but Kuhn liked her work, and so after high school, she worked in his office full time. She received additional training and functioned as a dental assistant for Kuhn, performing dental x-rays and making plaster of Paris molds.

One dental device of the period was the Cavitron ultrasonic cleaner. The Cavitron ultrasonic dental drill was first commercially produced in 1955 and then a more advanced Cavitron ultrasonic dental unit, which could be used for prophylaxis and cleaning, was released in 1957.[11] Until late 1965, the Cavitron was the only dental ultrasonic cleaner on the market.[12] The Cavitron Corporation was in Long Island City, Queens, New York.

Joan remembered that Larry had the Cavitron the whole time she helped with dental duties in his office. She did not use the machine herself because that duty was performed by the hygienists. She occasionally mentioned the Cavitron to Charlie in passing when discussing her work, and he was intrigued by it. In early 1962, Charlie decided that Larry would be his dentist. Kelman later wrote:

> Larry Kuhn was the dentist Joan was working for when I met her. When she introduced me to Larry, I immediately liked his sense of humor and his *joie de vivre*...[13]

Joan stopped working at Larry's office in January 1962 because she and Charlie were planning their wedding for April 1962. Joan recalled Larry joking to them that Charlie was "stealing" Joan away from his office.

Charlie recalled in his autobiography that he first saw a Cavitron at Larry's office. Joan recalled that Charlie asked to see Larry's Cavitron, and Larry did show it to Charlie. She believes this occurred much earlier than has been generally believed. In fact, she thought this demonstration of the Cavitron could have happened as early as 1962 (Fig. 5), but, as she did not witness it, she could not state precisely when it occurred. Some decades later, Larry recounted on film showing the Cavitron to Charlie (Fig. 6):

> I took him into the hygiene room. And I had just gotten in a new machine to clean teeth. It was an instrument like this that had various tips. He saw the way it vibrated at thousands of times per second, and saw the stream of water that cooled off the end of the tip. He saw it and he was elated.[14]

---

11 Cavitron Corp. v. Ultrasonic Research Corporation 1969.

12 Cavitron Corp. v. Ultrasonic Research Corporation 1969.

13 Kelman, 1985, p. 107.

14 Anker, 2010.

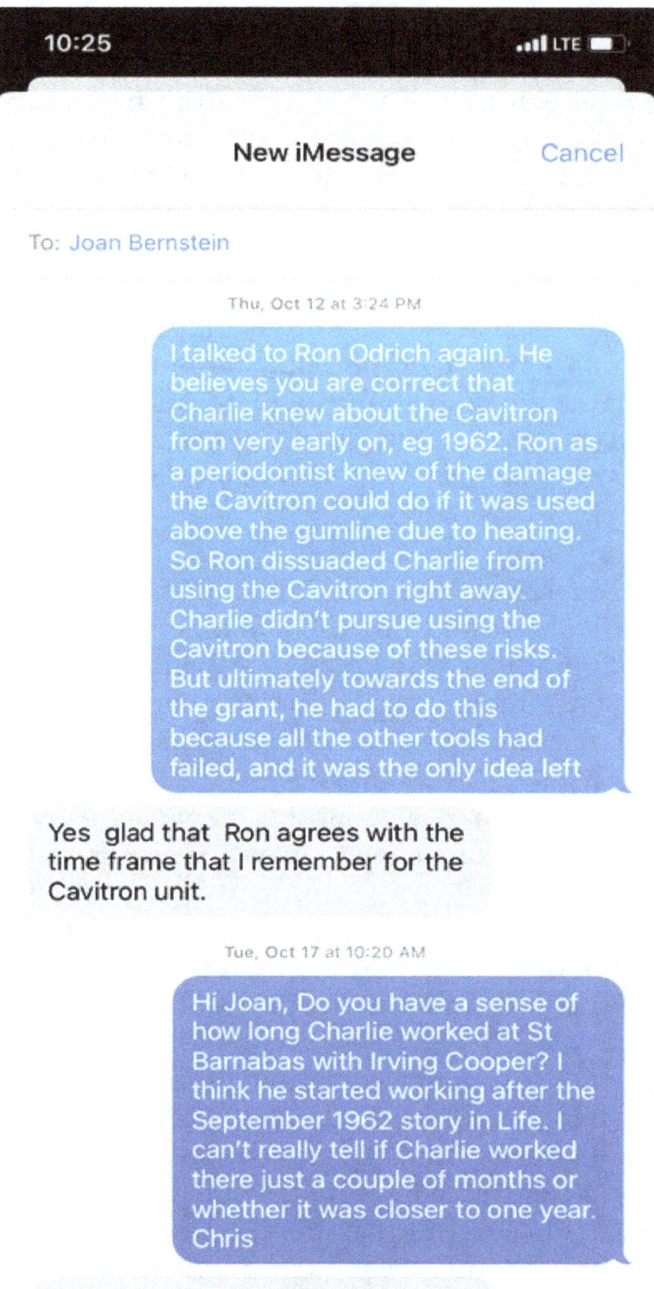



**Fig. 5.** Text message between Joan Bernstein and the author from October 12, 2023, confirming the interview indicating that Charles Kelman knew of the Cavitron in early 1962.

Larry continued to be the Kelman family dentist through the 1960s, at least for the children, as Joan remembered that he was able to handle their son David, who was difficult to examine as a young child, and their daughter Lesley remembers going to his office for her dental cleanings in the late 1960s. The Kuhn and Kelman families socialized on the holidays, and Joan would organize these get-togethers.

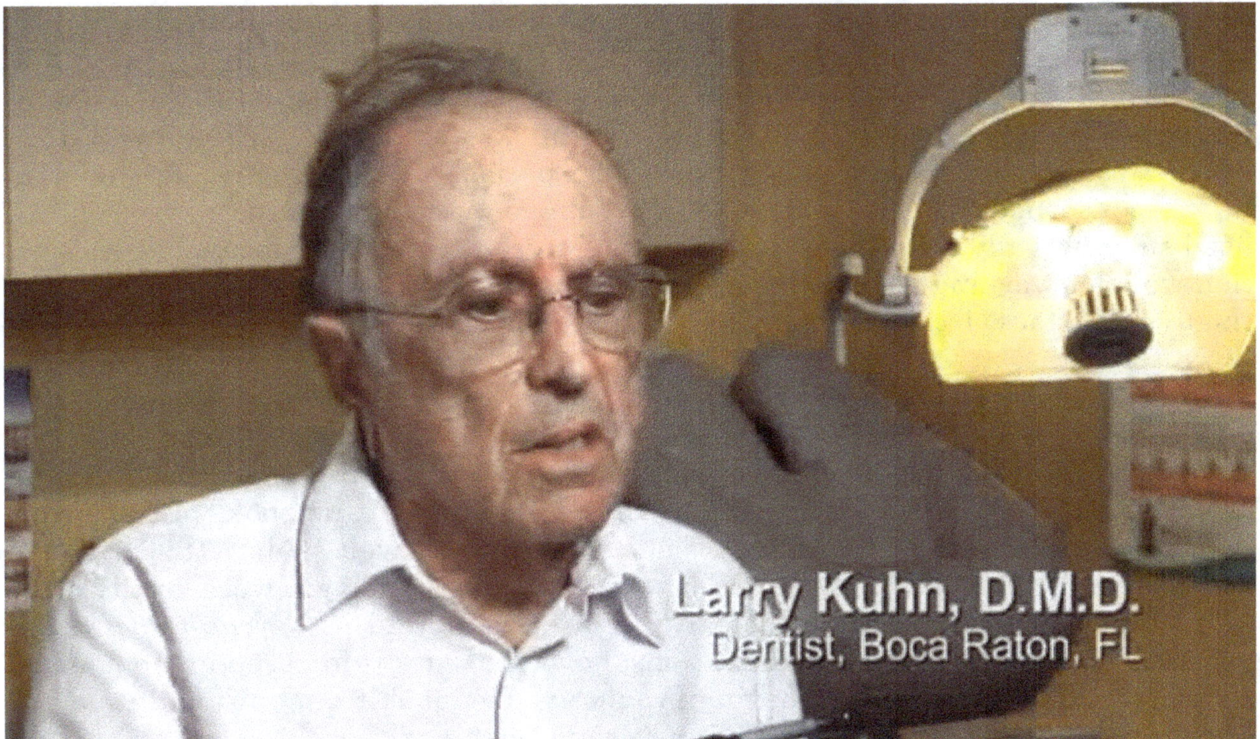


**Fig. 6.** Dentist Larry Kuhn recounting decades later how he showed Kelman the Cavitron (Anker 2010).

Another important person in Charlie's life in the 1960s was his friend, a periodontist and fellow jazz musician, Ronald B. Odrich. Odrich recalls that a fellow musician, Billy Costa, suggested they get in touch with each other because they had medicine and music in common. Odrich and Costa are both listed on the credits of a jazz album of "Bye Bye Birdie" by Bill Potts and his orchestra, the release of which was reported on Sep. 1, 1963, but Odrich remembered that he had known Costa since the 1950s. Like Kelman, Odrich played the clarinet and also the saxophone. In 1975, the *New York Times* called Odrich the best clarinet player in the United States. At Kelman's memorial, Odrich stated: "The very first time I met him…I knew I had a brother." Kelman and Odrich became close friends while Kelman worked at St. Barnabas Hospital in late 1962 or early 1963.[15]

Odrich had graduated from dental school in 1959 and then conducted 4 years of periodontal training. Both during his training and afterward, Odrich had a private

---

15 When dating the start of their friendship, it is helpful to recall that both Ron and Joan agree that Ron was not at the Kelman wedding in April 1962. Odrich remembers that Kelman was working with Irving Cooper at St. Barnabas Hospital in the Bronx when they met, because Odrich remembers wondering where that hospital was located. Odrich also remembers Kelman's disappointment when he left St. Barnabas under unfavorable circumstances. Kelman's St. Barnabas period was during the last quarter of 1962 and the first half of 1963.

practice in Manhattan.[16] Odrich remembered that Kelman visited him at his dental office not too long after they met because Odrich provided dental cleanings for Kelman around that time. Odrich recalled that as a medical man and future inventor, Kelman was always curious about all the dental devices in Ron's office. Ron did not have a Cavitron during Kelman's St. Barnabas period. As a prospective periodontist, he was concerned that the Cavitron could damage the root of the tooth, especially if used subgingivally, as some general dentists were performing. Because the irrigation was not working well in the early models, Ron felt the Cavitron was "cooking the tooth surface" if used subgingivally.

Kelman introduced Joan to his friend, songwriter Buddy Kaye, between their engagement in December 1961 and their wedding in April 1962.[17] Joan described Kaye as a "philosopher." Kelman wrote years later that Kaye introduced him to the book *Psycho-Cybernetics*, published in 1960, and that this book "put direction into my life."[18] *Psycho-Cybernetics* was written by Maxwell Maltz (1899-1975), a Jewish plastic surgeon from New York, who discusses his own work in the book. Many themes in Kelman's autobiography are also found in *Psycho-Cybernetics*: overcoming one's perceived imperfections, how creativity is fostered in moments of relaxation and "surrender," deriving productive feedback from one's failures, and how to handle emotional scars from one's relationships.[19]

## Cryotherapy for Retinal Detachments and Cataract Extraction (1962)

Kelman's first ophthalmic publications related to cryosurgery. Application of cold temperatures was first used in ophthalmology to produce chorioretinal inflammation by F. Schöler in 1918[20] and then to repair retinal detachments by Richard Deutschmann (1852–1935) of Hamburg and Giambattista Bietti (1907–1977) of Italy in 1933. Deutschmann had used solid carbon dioxide snow, and Bietti used this substance mixed with acetone.[21] It appears retinal cryotherapy was not widely adopted, however, and even Bietti used this procedure only rarely, because "its effect was milder than that obtained by diathermy."[22]

---

16 During his training, at least in the years 1960–1961, Odrich worked out of an office at 4 West 57th St. By 1963, and at least through 1966, he worked at 120 Central Park S. He remembers the office had a great view of Central Park.

17 Joan Bernstein, personal communication, Oct 25, 2023.

18 Kelman, 1991.

19 Maltz, 1960.

20 Schoeler, 1918. Was cited by Kelman AJO 1963, and by Garrison and Stockman, Index Medicus 1918, p. 471.

21 Rezaei & Abrams, 2005.

22 Bietti, 1950.

# 2. THE DEVELOPMENT OF SMALL INCISION CATARACT SURGERY

Bietti reviewed the retinal cryotherapy literature in June 1949, when he presented at the American Medical Association (AMA) meeting in Atlantic City. At this meeting, he presented his work on cryotherapy of the ciliary body by application of "solid carbon dioxide" to decrease aqueous production in glaucoma, which he had been begun developing during the War and had published in 1947.[23] Bietti's 1950 paper on cryotherapy of the ciliary body (which reviewed the retinal applicatons) was cited by notable figures, such as Kelman's professor Irving H. Leopold of the Wills Eye Hospital in 1957 and Conrad Berens of the New York Eye and Ear Infirmary in 1960.[24]

Cryoextraction of cataracts was first performed by Tadeusz Krwawicz of Lublin, Poland. He submitted his report on cryoextraction to the *British Journal of Ophthalmology* (*BJO*) on May 13, 1960, and it was published on April 1, 1961.[25] Krwawicz' work was noticed in America. David S. Johnson of the Boston University Medical Center saw Krwawicz' 1961 report in the *BJO* and wrote to him asking for a cryotherapy instrument, for which Johnson was willing to reimburse him. Johnson heard nothing for 1 year and thought that was the end of it, until in 1962, "the instrument, no longer than a fountain pen" arrived from Lublin (behind the "Iron Curtain") with a note from Krwawicz explaining that no payment was necessary. As Johnson experimented with the device in the laboratory "for more than a year," it was perhaps 1963 when he began using the device on patients with cataracts. By October 1964, Johnson had performed 70 cataract surgeries with Krwawicz' instrument at the Massachusetts Memorial Hospitals.[26] Johnson's work on cataract cryoextraction was described in the Medical Tribune on January 4, 1965 (Fig. 7).

Kelman learned that cryotherapy was being done in his area with a sophisticated cryoprobe by a neurosurgeon—Irving S. Cooper. Cooper had introduced major advances in neurosurgery, based, in part, on serendipity. In 1951, Cooper tied off the anterior choroidal artery during surgery because it was bleeding and fortuitously discovered that the patient's movement disorder was cured. He then set on a path to selectively destroy regions of the basal ganglia for various movement disorders, including localized chemical destruction. At Christmas in 1960, Cooper received as a Christmas gift a device, which would remove corks from bottles by injecting carbon dioxide. He became interested in how the injection of the gas produced localized cooling on his hand. A 1962 profile in *Look* magazine stated that this serendipitous

---

23 Bietti, 1950.

24 Scheie et al., 1955; Wudka & Leopold, 1957; Berens, 1960; Newell, 1993.

25 Krwawicz BJO, 1961. Krwawicz published a second report in Polish in 1961 (Krwawicz, Klinika Oczna 1961), which cited the BJO report. Krwawicz did not cite the retinal or glaucoma cryotherapy literature (Krwawicz BJO 1961; Krwawicz, Klinika Oczna 1961; Krwawicz, BJO 1963). Krwawicz' work was also described in the *Archives of Ophthalmology* by A. Ray Irvine of Los Angeles in a work submitted in January 1962, and published in April 1962.

26 Hickey, Oct 11, 1964.

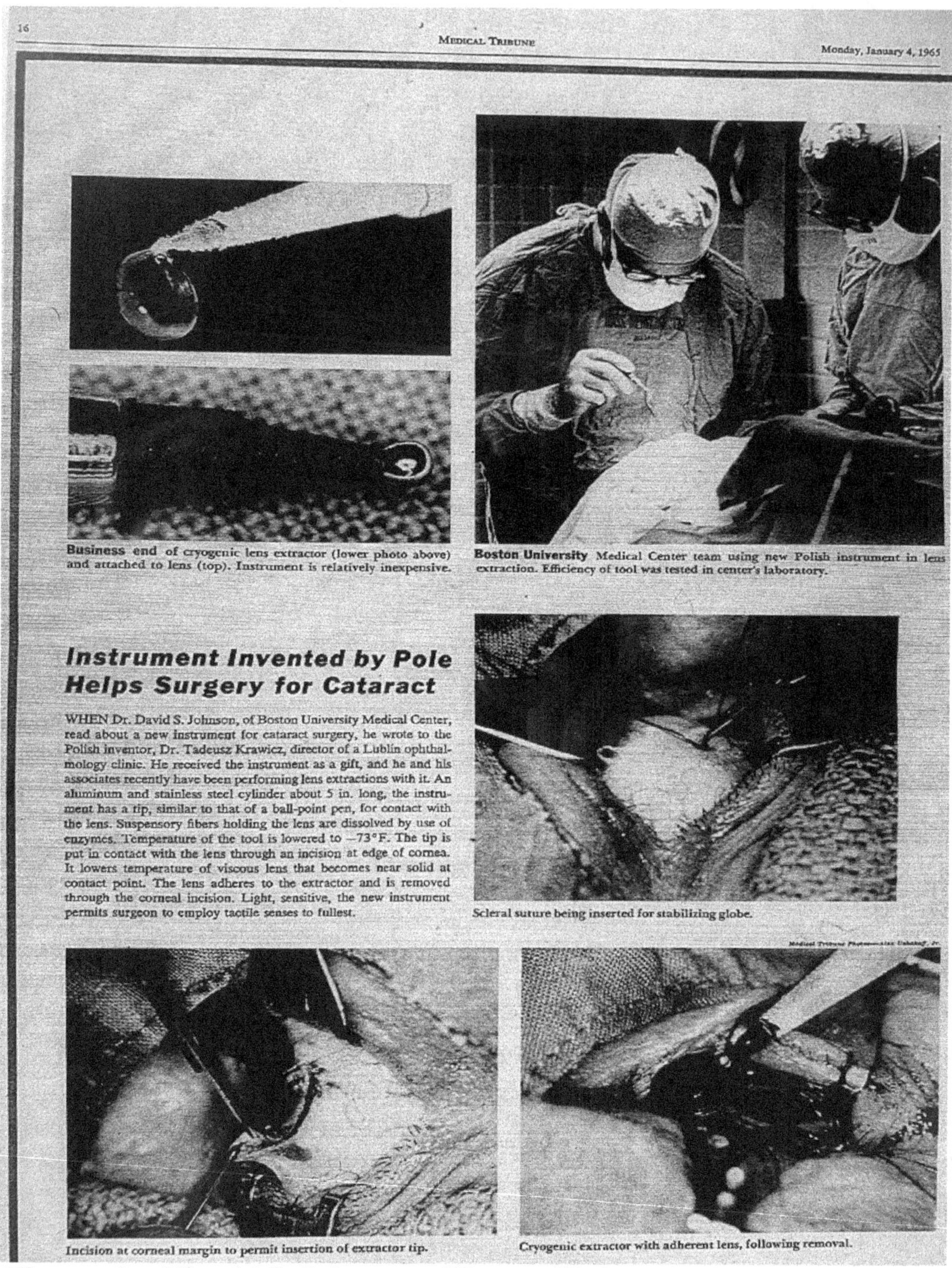

16     MEDICAL TRIBUNE     Monday, January 4, 1965

**Business end** of cryogenic lens extractor (lower photo above) and attached to lens (top). Instrument is relatively inexpensive.

**Boston University** Medical Center team using new Polish instrument in lens extraction. Efficiency of tool was tested in center's laboratory.

## Instrument Invented by Pole Helps Surgery for Cataract

WHEN Dr. David S. Johnson, of Boston University Medical Center, read about a new instrument for cataract surgery, he wrote to the Polish inventor, Dr. Tadeusz Krawicz, director of a Lublin ophthalmology clinic. He received the instrument as a gift, and he and his associates recently have been performing lens extractions with it. An aluminum and stainless steel cylinder about 5 in. long, the instrument has a tip, similar to that of a ball-point pen, for contact with the lens. Suspensory fibers holding the lens are dissolved by use of enzymes. Temperature of the tool is lowered to −73°F. The tip is put in contact with the lens through an incision at edge of cornea. It lowers temperature of viscous lens that becomes near solid at contact point. The lens adheres to the extractor and is removed through the corneal incision. Light, sensitive, the new instrument permits surgeon to employ tactile senses to fullest.

Scleral suture being inserted for stabilizing globe.

Incision at corneal margin to permit insertion of extractor tip.

Cryogenic extractor with adherent lens, following removal.

**Fig. 7.** The work of David S. Johnson of Boston University Medical Center on cataract cryoextraction was described in the Medical Tribune on January 4, 1965, page 16. This article, entitled "Instrument Invented by Pole…", was remembered by Kelman 20 years later when he wrote his autobiography. In fact, Kelman wrote that when his mentor, Irving Cooper, saw this article and realized that cryoextraction was performed in Poland before Kelman had performed the surgery, that Cooper fired Kelman on the spot. In fact, this article came out in January 1965, and Cooper fired Kelman from St. Barnabas Hospital in mid-1963. But, Kelman's recollection is accurate that Cooper was upset with Kelman for not properly crediting prior art, according to a phone call transcription from 1963.

event was the "origin" of his cryosurgical techniques.[27] On April 1, 1961, Cooper began using cryotherapy as a treatment for Parkinson.[28]

When Harvey A. Lincoff and John M. McLean of the New York Hospital-Cornell Medical Center presented on cryotherapy for retinal detachments in 1963, they stated: "In our first experiments, starting in the Spring of 1962, solid carbon dioxide applicators of various types were used." They are not specific about what these earliest experiments entailed, but clearly this group was trying to receive credit for initiating the renaissance in retinal cryotherapy.[29]

The summer of 1962 saw Cooper's work attracting national attention in both medical journals and the lay press. Cooper had performed "cryothalamectomy" in 100 patients with Parkinson between April 1, 1961, and April 1, 1962, and presented his outcomes at the AMA meeting in Chicago on June 28, 1962.[30] Cooper held a press conference at the AMA, his work was picked up by national newspapers, and he described the impact as a "bombshell."[31]

Kelman later recounted going to a national ophthalmology meeting in Chicago around the time he learned of Cooper's cryotherapy work.[32] Perhaps, it was this AMA meeting where Cooper presented his work, given that the AMA had an ophthalmology section.[33]

Cooper's neurosurgical cryotherapy was featured in two national pictorial news magazines in mid-1962: *Look* and *Life*. Joan told me the Kelman family did not subscribe to either of these. They subscribed to *Time*.

Later, Kelman recounted learning about Cooper's cryosurgery work in *Look* magazine while his wife dressed for a party (Fig. 8).[34] Kelman wrote:

---

27  Smothers, 1977.

28  Cooper, 1962. Cooper's efforts were picked up by an Associated Press wire story nationally on August 30, 1961, when he presented his results at the American Congress of Physical Medicine and Rehabilitation held in Cleveland. Cooper had performed fewer than a dozen of the cryosurgeries at that point ("Brain Tissue Frozen in Surgical Technique," Columbus Evening Dispatch, Aug. 31, 1961; Associated Press, Freezing technique, Utica Observer-Dispatch, Aug 30, 1961).

29  Lincoff, 1964. This presentation was at the Academy of Ophthalmology meeting in New York held Oct. 20-25, 1963.

30  Cooper, JAMA, Aug 18, 1962. Cooper's report was published on August 18, 1962.

31  Cooper, 1981, p. 237.

32  Kelman, 1985, p. 64.

33  Kelman, 1985, pp. 64-65. Kelman wrote that it was the Academy of Ophthalmology and Otolaryngology meeting, but the meeting for that organization was held in Las Vegas in 1962, not Chicago.

34  Fields, Daily News, May 18, 1965.

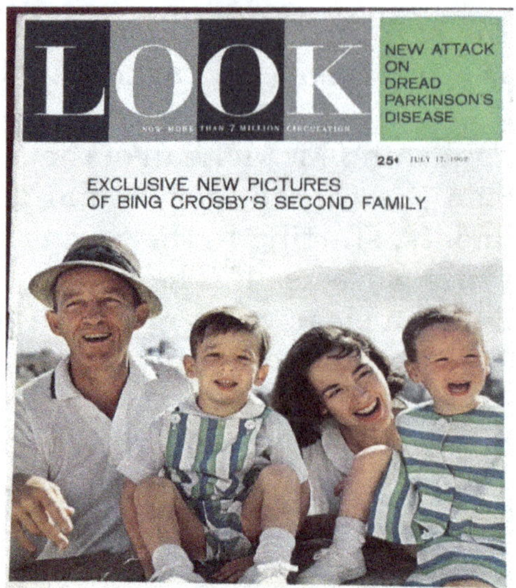


**Fig. 8.** *Look* magazine of July 17, 1962, featuring the cryosurgical work of Irving Cooper for Parkinson disease.

On the cover of the magazine was a picture of a man in a surgeon's mask. The story inside said the man—Dr. Irving S. Cooper—had found a way to cure victims of certain neurological diseases, such as Parkinson's, by freezing a tiny part of their brain. He had invented the technique and developed an apparatus which, at his command, would create a small ice ball at the tip of a slender probe placed deep inside the skull.[35]

Indeed, the July 17, 1962, *Look* magazine cover advertised the story "New Attack on Dread Parkinson's Disease," about Dr. Irving S. Cooper at St. Barnabas Hospital.[36]

*Life* magazine of September 14, 1962, featured on the cover a masked surgeon operating for its cover story of "One Hundred of the Most Important Young Men and Women in the United States (Fig. 9). The Take-Over Generation." The story noted that "Irving S. Cooper, [Age] 40. For 10 years, he has pioneered in the treatment of Parkinson's disease, developed the promising new cryogenic operation, a major breakthrough." (Fig. 10)[37]

At the start of my first conversation with Joan, I asked her the open-ended question: "Can you tell me about Charlie's research?" She responded immediately that Charlie got interested in cryosurgery when he saw Cooper featured in *Life* magazine. She never heard him speak about cryosurgery before that. Joan said she brought the *Life* magazine home because she was taking classes at New York University, and that magazine featured the president of New York University. Immediately after

---

35  Kelman, 1985, p. 61.

36  Moskin & Karales, 1962.

37  *Life.* Sep. 14, 1962.

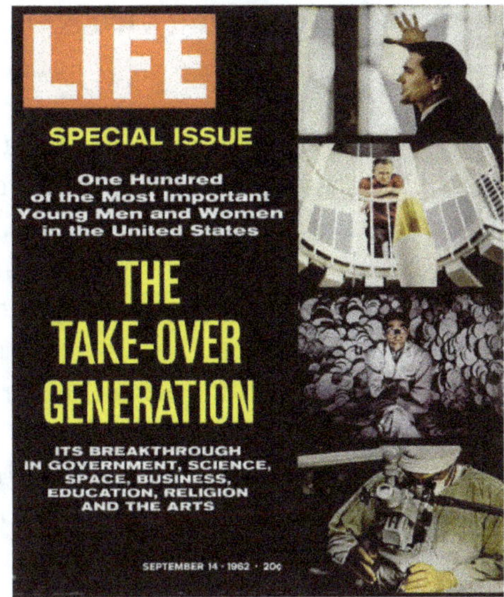

**Fig. 9.** *Life* magazine of September 14, 1962, featuring the cryosurgical work of Irving Cooper for Parkinson disease.

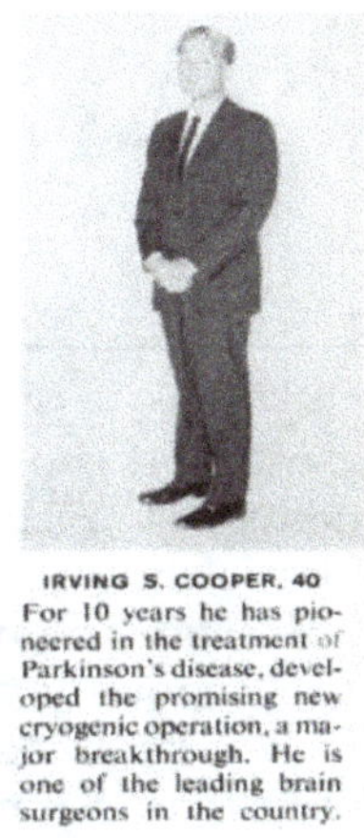



**Fig. 10.** Irving Cooper featured in *Life* magazine of September 14, 1962.

my phone call with Joan, I looked in the *Life* magazine to see if it really featured the president of New York University. Indeed, the 38-year-old James M. Hester was profiled. Joan remembered this September 14, 1962, *Life* magazine with the profile of Irving S. Cooper after 61 years!

It is not every day that a young doctor is glowingly featured in national news magazines and so it would be expected that the 40-year-old Cooper would keep a copy of both magazines in his lab, where Kelman could have seen them after Cooper hired him. The *Life* and *Look* features must have reinforced for the 32-year-old ophthalmologist that he was on the right track and might someday receive the same types of accolades that the 40-year-old Cooper was receiving. Cooper serendipitously learned that arterial occlusion could benefit movement disorders and that household devices to chill wine could also chill biological tissues. The themes in Cooper's biography, innovation through serendipitous discovery, would ultimately feature in Kelman's biography.

When Kelman saw the price of the cryotherapy machine, he knew he would need to use Cooper's machine. Kelman attempted to contact Cooper, by telephone, by telegram, and ultimately by maintaining a vigil in Cooper's waiting room. When they finally met, Cooper told him: "Kelman, you are the most persistent son of a bitch I ever met."[38] Joan remembers that their meeting was not too long after the *Life* magazine profile. Kelman stated that Cooper hired him on the spot to research ophthalmic cryotherapy, using Cooper's laboratory and personnel one morning per week.[39]

Joan's recollection is that right from the start, Charlie's interest in cryosurgery was to improve cataract surgery. This recollection is bolstered by a December 2, 1963, phone call between the administrator of the John A. Hartford Foundation, E. Pierre Roy, and Cooper. Roy's call notes indicate that "Dr. Kelman is not affiliated with Saint Barnabas Hospital and was only granted special privileges when he advanced the principal of cryosurgery for cataractous lens removal."[40] Kelman later wrote that he worked on cataract cryoextraction within the first 8 hours of starting in Cooper's lab.[41]

---

38  Kelman, 1985, p. 63.

39  Jacobson, 1984, p. 147. Kelman also wrote that the day after Cooper hired him, Kelman flew out to Chicago for the "American Academy of Ophthalmology" meeting (Kelman, 1985, p. 64). Kelman recalled that at this meeting, he felt like a nobody at the back of the auditorium and wanted to come up with an important discovery that would place him on the podium. Kelman recalled in his autobiography that at the Academy meeting, his colleagues probably had no idea about cryotherapy, and he actually left the meeting early to go work on cryotherapy. It is hard to explain this very vivid memory. The American Academy of Ophthalmology and Otolaryngology meeting was held in Chicago the previous year, from October 8–13, 1961 (Hughes, 1962). The 1962 meeting was held from November 4–9, 1962, in Las Vegas (Newell, 1962), and the October 1963 meeting was in New York (Report on Meetings 1964). It is conceivable that Kelman was thinking of the Section on Ophthalmology, 111th Annual Meeting of the American Medical Association, Chicago, June 26, 1962 (American Medical Association, Transactions 1962, p. 108). This was the same meeting at which Cooper presented his neurosurgical cryotherapy results. But this meeting still predates the July 17, 1962, *Look* magazine article about Cooper, and so Kelman's memory is hard to reconcile with known meetings. Kelman's involvement in Cooper's lab is confirmed as starting in the fall of 1962, because Kelman wrote in his grant of November 1963 that he "has worked at St. Barnabas Hospital for one year with Dr. Irving S. Cooper" (Hartford Foundation Files, Grant, Nov. 1963).

40  John A. Hartford Foundation records, 1963-1972.

41  Kelman, 1985, pp. 67-72. Kelman wrote that shortly after his first successful cataract cryoextraction surgery in a patient, Cooper submitted a photograph of the frozen cataract ("ice ball") produced by Kelman to the Hartford Foundation, which included the image in their "monthly newsletter." Jacobson (1984, p. 148) wrote that the photo of Kelman's "ice ball" was in the John A. Hartford Foundation Annual Report for 1962 (rather than the monthly newsletter). In 2023, the foundation archivist perused the annual report at my request and did not see anything about eye surgery.

While in Cooper's lab, Kelman also performed animal experiments related to retinal cryotherapy:

> I wanted to freeze the retina of the eye, creating an irritation there, which would make it form a firm scar to the underlying tissue.[42]

Whereas the predominant techniques at that time had used hot needles to produce a scar, the heat could damage the sclera, and Kelman believed that cryotherapy would spare the sclera and performed retinal cryotherapy in cats.[43]

Kelman wrote later that his article on cryotherapy for retinal detachment (in cats) and cryoextraction of cataracts (in humans) was rejected by a major ophthalmology journal.[44] Kelman suspected that the journal reviewers might have appropriated his ideas. Cooper told Kelman he should focus on cataracts and leave the retinal work to the retinal specialists at a nearby medical school.[45] Timing-wise, the Cornell group of Lincoff and McClean later presented that they had received the type of probe used by Cooper and manufactured by the Linde Division of Union Carbide in November 1962.[46]

Ophthalmologist Adolph Posner, of New York, who hailed originally from Poland, helped Kelman get his cryosurgery paper published in *Eye, Ear, Nose & Throat Monthly* in January 1963.[47] Kelman's article referred to retinal detachment in the title and indicated that he thought of the idea of cryotherapy for retinal detachment. In contrast, cataract cryoextraction was only mentioned as a side note and was described as an existing technology. As first author, Kelman seems to have been aware that others were performing cataract cryoextraction by January 1963.

Kelman and Cooper submitted a second report on cataract cryoextraction, which was accepted for publication in the *American Journal of Ophthalmology* on May 20, 1963.[48] In this report, Kelman cited prior retinal and cataract cryosurgery work.

---

42 Kelman, 1985, pp. 61-62.

43 Kelman, 1985, p. 66.

44 Kelman, 1985, pp. 74-76.

45 Kelman, 1985, pp. 74-76.

46 Lincoff, 1964.

47 Kelman, EENT Monthly, 1963. Kelman and Cooper in EENT Monthly 1963 cited Cooper's neurosurgical work, but no ophthalmic cryotherapy papers. Kelman, 1991. Cooper later wrote: "In collaboration with a young man who had just finished his residency in ophthalmology, Dr. Charles Kelman, I investigated cryogenic ophthalmic surgery, including the cryosurgery for retinal detachment and other ocular conditions, but particularly the cryosurgical removal of cataracts" (Cooper, 1981, p. 233). In January 1963, Krwawicz published a second article in the *British Journal of Ophthalmology* on his case series of cataract cryoextractions, and he also did not cite the earlier retinal cryopexy work from Europe (Krwawicz BJO, 1963).

48 Kelman AJO, 1963. Kelman and Cooper cited Schoeler, Deutschmann, Bietti, and Krwawicz. Kelman's professor Irving Leopold knew of Bietti's cryotherapy work, and was an editor of

Kelman developed an improved cryoprobe. His brother-in-law, Robert Dorfman, introduced him to Ralph Crump at Frigitronics, the company that manufactured the probe, which Kelman called a "cryostylet" for cataract removal.[49]

The October 1963 meeting of the Academy was a "coming out party" for ophthalmic cryotherapy in America. At the meeting, Kelman showed a film of his cryotherapy-induced retinal lesions in cats, as well as cryoextraction of cataracts in patients.[50]

Lincoff presented his work on retinal cryotherapy using the "Cooper-Linde cryosurgical unit for the treatment of parkinsonism, an apparatus that could deliver to the end of a probe a temperature ranging from +37°C to −180°C. The frozen tip of the probe could be disengaged from the tissues within a few seconds by raising the temperature. This made it possible to control both temperature and time of application in an effort to find the ideal therapeutic lesion for the treatment of retinal detachment." After experiments in animals, Lincoff developed for human subjects a probe smaller than the original Cooper neurosurgical probe. Lincoff's probe began to be used in patients in February 1963.[51]

In the discussion that followed Lincoff's paper, Edward W. D. Norton of Miami stated that with respect to recent advances in retinal detachment therapy:

> Today we have heard of the application of cold to ophthalmic tissues and, as pointed out by Dr. Lincoff, we again are borrowing from the past. This should emphasize to the young investigator the importance of searching the literature, especially the foreign literature, before he reports his 'new' discovery...I saw Dr. Kelman's motion picture yesterday for the first time and would prefer not to spend much time discussing it.[52]

Norton believed that cryoextraction of cataracts could be useful for dislocated lenses and that its role could expand if better instrumentation were available. Kelman was essentially getting called out for not reading the literature, and this must have been a very public humiliation.

At the October 1963 meeting, R. David Sudarsky of the Manhattan Eye, Ear, and Throat Hospital presented a liquid nitrogen–based cryosurgical probe useful for both cataract and retinal surgeries in October 1963.[53] Ultimately, Sudarsky's cryoprobe came to be favored over that of Kelman in the marketplace.

---

the journal.

49  Kelman, 1991; Kelman, 1966, p. viii.

50  Kelman & Cooper "Cryophthalmic," 1964.

51  Lincoff, 1964.

52  Lincoff, 1964.

53  Sudarsky, 1963.

It should be noted that cryoextraction of cataracts and small incision surgery were not necessarily totally separate projects in Kelman's mind. The goal of small incision surgery is to somehow make the cataract smaller. In his January 1963 publication on ophthalmic cryosurgery, Kelman devoted only five sentences to cataracts. One of those sentences noted that freezing "aids in the rupture of the zonules by causing a shrinkage of the lens."[54] By November 18, 1963, Kelman noted in his Hartford Foundation grant application, specifically in the context of small incision cataract surgery: "I have found that freezing a lens shrinks it considerably." As we see later, this November 1963 proposal also discussed freezing the lens, moving it to the anterior chamber, thawing it out, and then breaking it into pieces. In other words, cryosurgery could be part of a small incision approach. Indeed, Joan recalls that right from the start, Charlie was interested in cryoextraction of cataracts because it could facilitate small-incision surgery.

In his autobiography, Kelman recalls that Cooper fired him from the St. Barnabas Hospital and that this was a major setback. Odrich agreed that Kelman was "devastated" by this firing. Presumably, this would have occurred between May 20, 1963, when their joint publication on cryoextraction was accepted, and November 18, 1963, when Kelman submitted a solo grant to the Hartford Foundation. On December 2, 1963, E. P. Roy of the Hartford Foundation called Cooper for a reference and recorded: "Dr. Cooper questions his scientific integrity in regard to acknowledging the work of others in the field and also support of his past work...they were planning to establish a Department of Ophthalmology at Saint Barnabas Hospital emphasizing the cryogenic surgery, but Dr. Kelman would not be asked to participate."[55]

## Chemical Dissolution of the Cataract (1963)

Kelman later wrote that in 1963, just before he received funding from the Hartford Foundation (which we know to have occurred in January 1964), he worked for 1 year to try to emulsify the lens using chemical or enzymatic means.[56] There certainly was precedent for the use of enzymatic dissolution of intraocular tissues in ophthalmology. By May of 1957, Barraquer of Spain had pioneered lenticular zonulolysis with chymotrypsin.[57] If Kelman did work on chemical dissolution of cataracts, these efforts were likely perfunctory. Neither Joan nor Ron Odrich remembered such efforts. The only tangentially related mention I could in the Foundation files was a letter from Kelman from March 20, 1969, which simply states regarding hyphema that "Enzymatic dissolution of the blood clot is at best, erratically successful", but this

---

54 Kelman EENT, 1963.

55 Hartford Foundation files, 1963-1972.

56 Kelman, 1970; Kelman "History," 1974; Kelman AJO, 1967. None of the 400 pages in the Hartford Foundation file covering work on the grant from January 1964 to 1972 relate to chemical dissolution lens. If he worked on this during the grant period, either it was at a low level, or he did not want to apprise the foundation.

57 Harris, 1961.

could have related to the ophthalmic work by others, as he mentioned it to justify his study of phacoemulsification for hyphema.

But where could Kelman have done such work? It is conceivable that Kelman could have experimented with chemical dissolution while in Cooper's lab at St. Barnabas. Cooper, after all, had used absolute alcohol for chemical destruction of the basal ganglia. Kelman seems to have been still affiliated with Cooper at St. Barnabas on May 20, 1963, when their second paper on ophthalmic cryotherapy was accepted for publication.[58]

Moreover, Kelman began research at Manhattan Eye, Ear, Nose,and Throat Hospital in the second half of 1963, which he self-funded, according to his November 1963 grant.[59]

## Small Incision Cataract Surgery on the Hartford Grant (1964)

On November 18, 1963, Kelman applied for a grant from the John A. Hartford Foundation, and the program started on January 15, 1964 (Figure 11). Kelman had the support of E. Pierre "Pete" Roy, who had worked as administrator for the John A. Hartford Foundation since 1952. Roy was a trained accountant and had gotten the job at the Foundation because he was skilled at spotting financial impropriety when working for the A&P grocery chain.[60] In this grant, Kelman indicated that he had also applied for an NIH grant for the same research, but that he would not hear about the NIH grant until March 1964, and if the Foundation funded his work, he would not take NIH funding.

Kelman's plan was broad in scope, covering congenital cataracts, ocular oncology, glaucoma, and retinal detachment repair. But ultimately the most important proposal was the second to last: "a new technique for surgical removal of a cataractous

---

58 Kelman & Cooper AJO, 1963.

59 A June 17, 1963, letter from Thurston H. Long, the hospital administrator stated: "At a meeting...it was noted that you now have specialty boards. The Board of Surgeon Directors has therefore endorsed your promotion to Assistant Attending Surgeon... In the light of your expected promotion, it is expected that the cryosurgery which you propose to do will be scheduled after July 1st... Meanwhile, and before any work is started, it is requested that you present a documented research protocol to the Hospital's research committee, of which Dr. Herbert Katzin is the Eye member." A press release from the Manhattan Eye, Ear, and Throat Hospital dated October 23, 1963, described his presentation at the Academy and stated: "...Doctor Kelman is beginning a cryosurgical (freezing) program of investigation into many branches of eye disease at Manhattan Eye, Ear and Throat Hospital." A November 29, 1963, letter from Herbert M. Katzin, MD, head of the research committee and head of the eye bank at Manhattan Eye, Ear, and Throat Hospital recommending Kelman to the Hartford Foundation stated "...Dr. Kelman is in every way I know competent in his work, both as an ophthalmologist and as one to carry on research" (Hartford Foundation files, 1963-1972).

60 Jacobson, 1984, pp. 19-27.

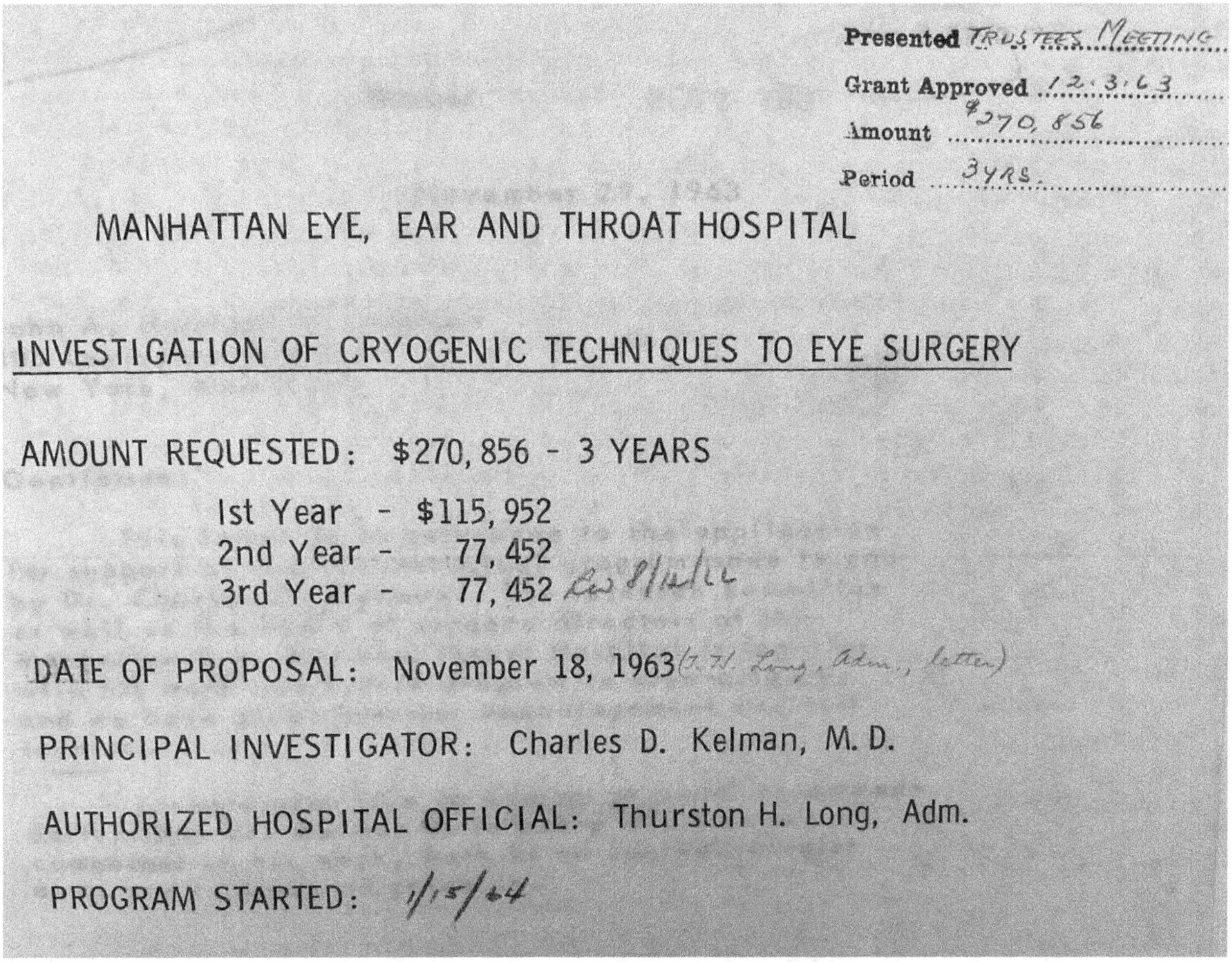

Presented *TRUSTEES MEETING*
Grant Approved *12.3.63*
Amount *$270,856*
Period *3 YRS.*

MANHATTAN EYE, EAR AND THROAT HOSPITAL

INVESTIGATION OF CRYOGENIC TECHNIQUES TO EYE SURGERY

AMOUNT REQUESTED:   $270,856 - 3 YEARS

      Ist Year   -   $115,952
      2nd Year  -     77,452
      3rd Year   -     77,452

DATE OF PROPOSAL:  November 18, 1963 *(T. H. Long, Adm., letter)*

PRINCIPAL INVESTIGATOR:  Charles D. Kelman, M. D.

AUTHORIZED HOSPITAL OFFICIAL:  Thurston H. Long, Adm.

PROGRAM STARTED:  *1/15/64*

**Fig. 11.** Kelman's grant application covering small incision cataract surgery, starting January 15, 1964 (Hartford Foundation files, 1963–1972).

lens that will require a hospital stay of twenty-four hours instead of two weeks and a return to normal activity within one week instead of two weeks and a return to normal activity within one week instead of thirty days" (Fig. 12).[61]

As noted earlier, freezing the lens was felt to assist with small incision cataract surgery. Kelman wrote:

> I have found that freezing a lens shrinks it considerably. I intend to develop a method of cataract extraction which may be performed through an extremely small opening in the eye, necessitating perhaps only one suture, if any, and removing this lens through the small opening described. This would immeasurably reduce the convalescence period of the patient and if this technique proves possible, will be a major step forward in cataract surgery.[62]

---

61  Kelman, Nov. 18, 1963, Hartford grant proposal.
62  Kelman, Nov 18, 1963 grant.

The proposed investigation will include development of cryosurgery for
(1) early removal of congenital cataracts, a major source of loss of
vision in children, which cannot be performed by conventional techniques
until after the age of six years when the strong adhesion of the lens
to the vitreous body normally subsides--at this late a date complications frequently have already permanently impaired the eyesight (2) de-
termining whether a tumor in the posterior portion of the eye is benign
or malignant, this is now not possible and when tumors are detected the
entire eye is usually enucleated as a precautionary measure (3) treatment
of glaucoma by permanently restoring the ductile drainage of aqueous
fluid for relief of ocular pressure, a factor which eventually causes
blindness (4) a new technique for surgical removal of a cataractous
lens that will require a hospital stay of twenty-four hours instead of
two weeks and a return to normal activity within one week instead of
thirty days (5) improved cryosurgery for repairing retinal detachment.

**Fig. 12.** Scope of Kelman's grant application covering small incision cataract surgery, starting January 15, 1964 (Hartford Foundation files, 1963–1972).

the eye.  The lens will be allowed to thaw and resume its normal

consistency.  A needle will be introduced into the eye and the

cataract will be punctured.  The contents of the cataract, along

with the capsule, will be aspirated through this previously made

small incision, by using a special two-way syringe.  This procedure

**Fig. 13.** Idea for cataract aspiration with a needle in Kelman's grant application
covering small incision cataract surgery, starting January 15, 1964 (Hartford Foundation files, 1963–1972).


The first idea was to use cryoextraction to dislocate the lens into the anterior
chamber, where it would be thawed, and then aspirated with a special needle, in
the manner similar to what medieval Arabic authors had attempted (Figure 13).

A second idea was to thaw the lens in the anterior chamber, as before, and then
macerate the lens within a bag (Fig. 14).

Interestingly, Kelman's annual progress reports were divided into a report about
small incision surgery, marked "Confidential," and a separate report covering all
other aspects of ophthalmic cryotherapy. Kelman wrote a progress report on the
small incision surgery, which was stamped "received" by the Hartford Foundation
on April 19, 1965. The report was marked "Confidential," and I found it next to
another confidential report in the Kelman file collection addressed to E. P. Roy,
the director. The "confidential" progress reports on small incision surgery did not

troducing through the small incision, a plastic bag to enclose the cataract, with the mouth of the bag protruding through the incision. The cataract will then be macerated within the plastic bag and the plastic bag along with the macerated cataract will be extracted through the small opening. These procedures, if successful, would permit almost immediate mobilization of the patient and would eliminate the necessity of keeping a postoperative cataract in the hospital for more than 24 hours. It would enable the patient to return to work possibly within one week.

**Fig. 14.** Idea for cataract maceration within a bag in Kelman's grant application covering small incision cataract surgery, starting January 15, 1964 (Hartford Foundation files, 1963–1972).

mention Kelman's name or the Manhattan Eye, Ear, and Throat Hospital. In parallel, there were separate progress reports received April 19, 1965, and from April 5, 1966, which mentioned Kelman's name and the Manhattan Eye, Ear, and Throat Hospital. These progress reports were not labeled "confidential" and were related to all aspects of ophthalmic cryotherapy (except small incision surgery). (Fig. 15)

In the confidential April 19, 1965 report, after reiterating the benefits of small incision surgery, including reduced hospitalization time, the report stated:

During this past year, much time, effort and thought has gone into solution of this problem. Several dozen instruments have been designed, built, and tried during this time...A small instrument has been devised and now works very well, which can enter the eye through a 1 1/2 mm. incision, grasp the lens, and partially dislocate it. Another instrument has been devised which enters the eye through a second small incision 180° away from the first, and while the first instrument is holding the lens, can safely be used to rupture the zonules over an area of 90 degrees. An instrument has been devised and is presently being modified which will be able to support the lens from behind and encapsulate it into a small silicon bag.

These instruments represent a few successful ones out of the many, many instruments devised and tried. To speed up development of this technique...an instrument maker and designer will be hired fulltime to work on this project with me. This person has an extensive background in the field of research development and instrument making, and has already, on a part-time basis, been more successful than any other instrument maker I have used. Once the problem of slipping the lens into the bag has

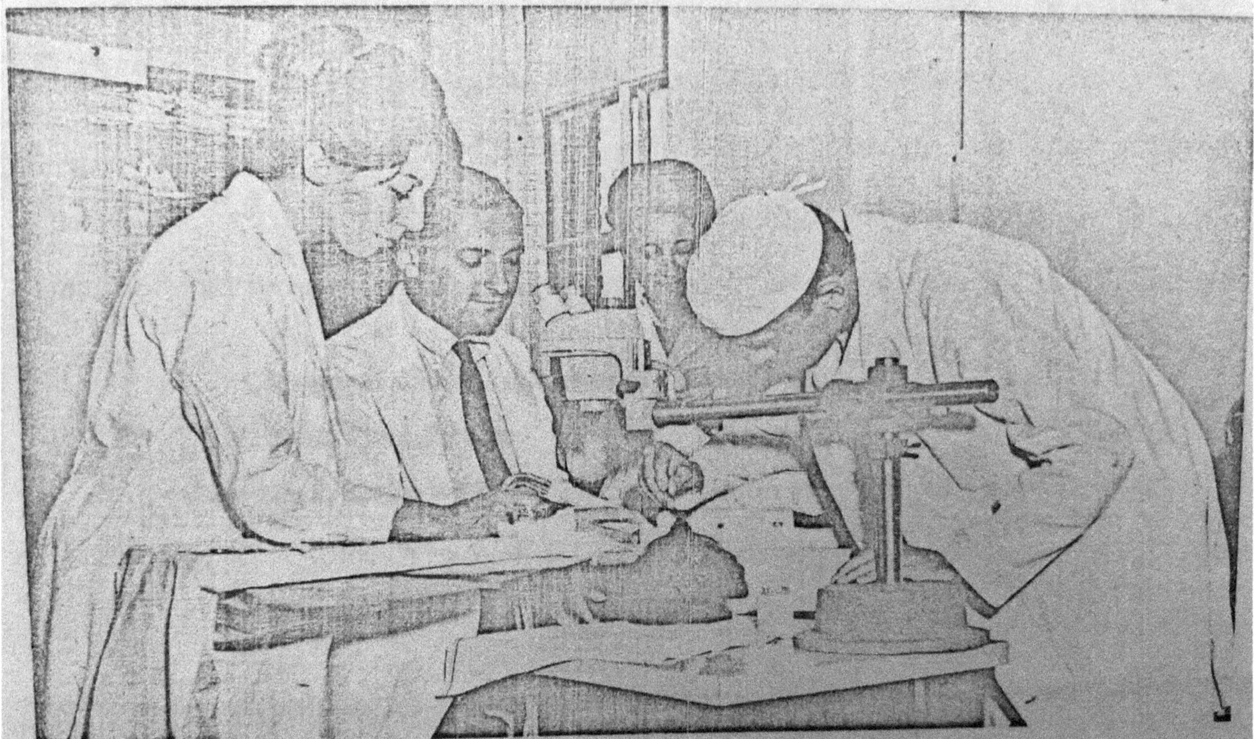



CRYOSURGERY RESEARCH at Manhattan Eye, Ear and Throat is a team effort. Assistant attending surgeon Charles D. Kelman, M.D., second from left, the Hospital's director of cryosurgery research, is pictured with his "team-mates" Miss Sheila Watson, Mrs. Kety Sapounova, and William Rice.

**Fig. 15.** Charles Kelman performing cryosurgery research with Sheila Watson RN (nurse), Kety Sapoenova (histology technician), and William Rice (coordinator), featured in the Hartford Courant on November 12, 1964 in an article entitled "Hartford Hospital Performs Successful Eye Surgery Using Freezing Technique".

been solved, the remainder of the operation is easy. The lens is fragmented within the bag, and irrigated from the bag. Then, the practically empty bag is withdrawn through one of the tiny incisions, and the operation is finished.[63]

---

63  Hartford foundation files, 1963-1972.

# Start of the Phacoemulsification Program (by February 1965)

In February 1965, Kelman began working with Anton Banko, an engineer and researcher at Cavitron, to develop ultrasonic phacoemulsification,[64] even though the April 1965 reports to the Foundation did not mention this development. This starting date for the work with Cavitron comes from lecture notes written by Banko (Fig. 16).[65]

ANTON BANKO

PHAKO FRAGMENTATION

THE PHAKOEMULSIFICATION PROJECT STARTED IN FEBRUARY 1965 ...

**Fig. 16.** Lecture notes written by engineer Anton Banko indicate that Banko and Kelman began working on phacoemulsification in February 1965. Banko indicated in the notes that he revised them in 1985, so they were presumably originally written before that year.

This initiation of the formal research program was preceded by two events: (1) the idea to use the Cavitron for cataract surgery and (2) an initial test of the Cavitron in an animal eye. The timing of these two prior events is uncertain.

When Kelman was posthumously awarded the Lasker medal in 2004, the Lasker Foundation stated that the epiphany that the Cavitron could be used for cataract surgery occurred at a dentist's office in 1964 (Goldstein 2004). The date of 1964 is certainly plausible. Joseph Goldstein of the Lasker Foundation indicated in an email to me in 2024 that the determination that the year was 1964 came from communication with Kelman's colleagues. It is unclear to what degree this determination was based on inside information which ultimately derived from Kelman, and to what degree it was based on interpretation of Kelman's writings, which included an incorrect date for the grant.

Charlie wrote in his autobiography that the epiphany that the Cavitron could be used for cataract surgery first came about at Larry's dental office. Larry's son had also been told by his father that the two were together when the idea came about. Perhaps that is true.

---

64 Allen, 1995.

65 Anton Banko's lecture notes from 1985 were kindly provided by his son, William Banko. In addition, an advertisement for the Heslin-Mackool Ocusystem, developed by Banko, and advertised in July 1980, contained a photo of Banko and stated: "In 1965, the Phacoemulsifier was designed and co-invented by Anton Banko and Dr. Charles Kelman."

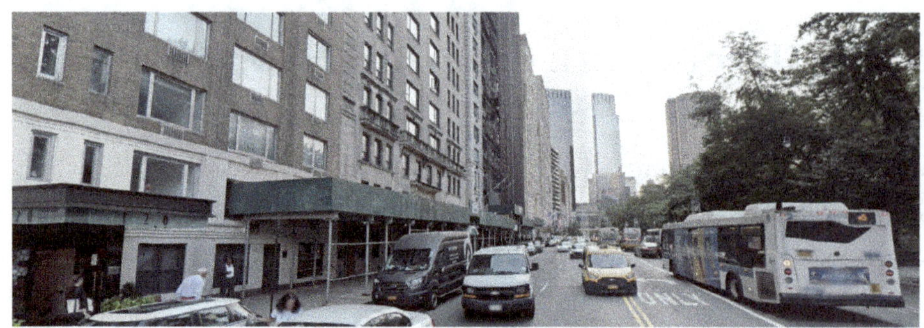

**Fig. 17.** Location of Ronald Odrich's dental practice at 120 Central Park South in Manhattan. Odrich practiced at this location from 1963 through at least 1966, based on dental directories of the period.

But some evidence would suggest that the epiphany came about at Ron Odrich's office (Fig. 17). First, Kelman's former resident and fellow from 1969 to 1973, Norman Medow, recalled that the entire story of Kelman thinking of the idea while having his teeth cleaned at the dentist, going to his lab to retrieve a cataract, and then returning to the dentist's office to test the Cavitron on the cataract all related to Ron Odrich. Dr. Medow states that Kelman frequently told him that the idea occurred to him at Odrich's office. Dr. Medow also knew Odrich's sons, Marc and Steven, who both became ophthalmologists. Dr. Medow told all of this to me (CTL) at the reception of the Cogan Society meeting on April 19, 2024, and provided his permission to publish these statements. Dr. Medow then repeated the statement that Kelman told him that he thought of the idea while at Odrich's dental office having his teeth cleaned, to the audience gathered for the Cogan Society meeting in the Bascom Palmer Eye Institute auditorium, during the comment period for my presentation about Kelman on April 20, 2024. In an email on June 6, 2024, Dr. Medow confirmed: "I was Charlie's Clinical Fellow 1972–1973.....He was doing Phaco regularly then on patients and was teaching it in weekly courses he held for interested Ophthalmologists who came to NYC for 5 days to learn phaco......I heard Charlie talk about his Epiphany at Dr. Odrich's office Many, Many times.....I also have heard the Odrich Brothers [Steven and Marc] speak about it as well....I did not know Ron Odrich but may have met him on occasion." Medow further explained that he "1st met the Odrich Brothers when they were on staff at MEETH and when Marc was involved as a researcher in the early days of refractive Surgery.....they are both junior to me in age and I first met them as they arrived after I left fellowship..."

If the epiphany occurred at Odrich's office, this would also fit with Odrich's statements that Charlie visited his office for dental cleanings early in their relationship, when Odrich did not have a Cavitron, and that Charlie was very interested in all the devices in the dental office. One could imagine the two of them pondering the likelihood that each of the devices could be modified to perform cataract surgery. Either of them could have suggested the Cavitron, regardless of whether it was in Ron's office. Of course, Ron knew about the Cavitron as a periodontist. But, Kelman could also have known about the Cavitron, from talking to his wife, or because the Cavitron was featured on the front page of the New York Times on Feb. 9, 1963,

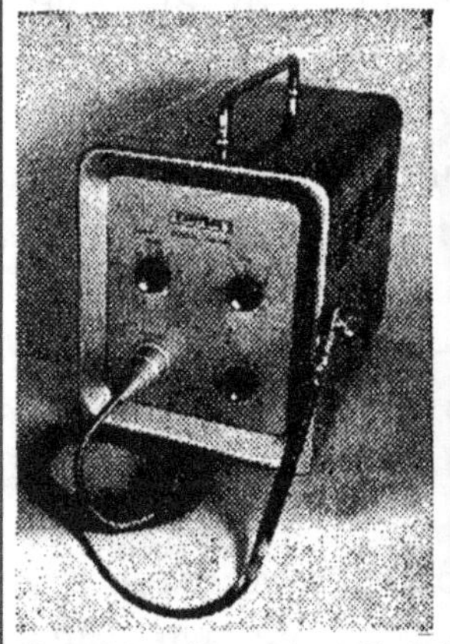
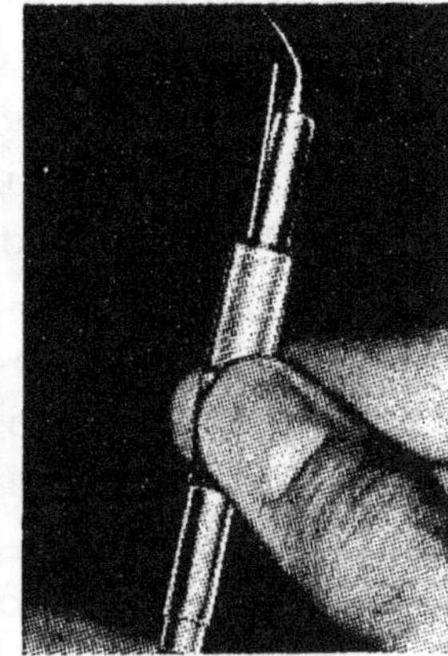

# Patented Ultrasonic Unit Cleans Teeth Painlessly

Complete ultrasonic unit, left, and close-up of handpiece

**By STACY V. JONES**
Special to The New York Times.

WASHINGTON, Feb. 8 — A New York company received a patent this week for an ultrasonic dental unit designed for the painless removal of tartar and stains. The dentist gently guides a tip vibrating 25,000 times a second under a spray of water.

The invention, called the Dentsply-Cavitron Unit, is now being widely distributed to dentists at about $800. It is manufactured by Cavitron Ultrasonics, Inc.

The patient who used to wince at the scraping of the old hand scalpel on his teeth can now relax, according to the company, under this superior method of prophylaxis. The cavitation (partial vacuum of the bubbles) is described as beneficial for the gums.

The generator steps up ordinary alternating current from 50 or 60 to 25,000 cycles. An energizing coil of wire around the tubular hand-piece causes a stack of metal strips to expand and contract one-thousandth of an inch. The movement, which is so rapid as to be beyond audible range, is transmitted to the tip.

The instrument was invented for the company by Dr. Claus Kleesattel, an ultrasonics engineer; Dr. Lewis Balamuth, head of research, and Arthur Kuris, head of engineering.

The patent (3,076,904) covers possible applications also to sur-

Continued on Page 12, Column 3

**Fig. 18.** On Feb. 9, 1963, the Cavitron prophylactic dental cleaner was featured on the front page of the New York Times, when the patent was granted.

when the patent for dental prophylaxis was granted (Fig. 18). If the idea to use the Cavitron for cataract surgery occurred to Kelman before Odrich had a Cavitron, this could explain why Kelman traveled all the way out to the far side of Queens to Larry's office to examine the Cavitron and test it for eye surgery.

Odrich did not state that the epiphany occurred at his office, but he came close. When I asked him on a phone call where he was when he first heard about the idea to use the Cavitron for eye surgery, he replied "I was in my office." In fact, he indicated that Kelman had the epiphany elsewhere, and then visited Odrich's office on the very same day, and they discussed the idea. Odrich indicated that he discouraged Charlie from this idea, because he thought that the Cavitron would thermally damage the eye. Both Charlie and Ron were concerned that irrigation to cool the device could increase the intraocular pressure. A few days later, Odrich emailed me to clarify that Kelman actually visited his office a few days after the epiphany, and they discussed it.

The first test of the Cavitron in an animal eye must have occurred when Charlie had access to a lab with animals (ie, after October 1962), and before February 1965. By most accounts (Charlie and Larry's comments to reporters and to his family), Charlie and Larry were together when this test was carried out.[66] The reporter who spoke to both Charlie and Larry indicated that the test was on the lens from a cat's eye.[67] Larry's son remembers that it was a test in an animal, and Charlie merely stated that it was a "cataract" from the hospital, which could also be consistent with a test in the cataract of a cat from a hospital laboratory. Indeed, Kelman specified that this test occurred when he worked in a laboratory.[68]

The initial test was unsuccessful. A reporter recounted from Larry's point of view: "The dentist watched intently as Kelman took the ultrasonic drill and applied it to the cataract. Nothing happened. The lens was pushed around a bit, but that was all."[69]

Larry Kuhn's son remembered that his father "went somewhere" to test the Cavitron for eye surgery. In addition, Kelman told the Saturday Review reporter in 1972 that after the failed test at Kuhn's office: "I went back to the laboratory discouraged but decided to give the reaction of cataracts to ultrasonic drills a closer look—under the microscope. What I saw convinced me. Larry Kuhn's drill did dissolve cataracts—not enough to be visible to the naked eye, but enough to make me realize the technique would work." Putting these two statements together, it seems possible that Larry accompanied Charlie back to his lab with the Cavitron to test its worth for eye surgery at the hospital.

Kelman had at least 2 years left on the Hartford Foundation grant when he began the formal research program with Cavitron. However, he was seriously feeling the pressure. In contrast with the rapid success Kelman had seen in the lab with ophthalmic cryotherapy, he had probably worked for several years on small incision surgery and had little to show for it. He describes in his autobiography feeling enormous pressure and worried about taking almost $300,000 and simply failing. Ron describes Charlie as "desperate" and "panicked" with "his back against the wall" at this point. Why did Charlie turn to the Cavitron? The process of elimination. Nothing else had worked. He was out of options. He had proven the risks of the alternatives. The Cavitron might have had risks—thermal injury—but perhaps he could manage them with adequate irrigation to cool the eye.

Charlie met with Robert (Bob) Navin, the president at Cavitron, about developing an ophthalmic phacoemulsifier. It was necessary to add suction to the dental probe

---

66 Vachon, 1972; Kelman, 1985; Anker, 2010.

67 Vachon, 1972.

68 Kelman, 1985; Vachon, 1972.

69 Vachon, 1972.

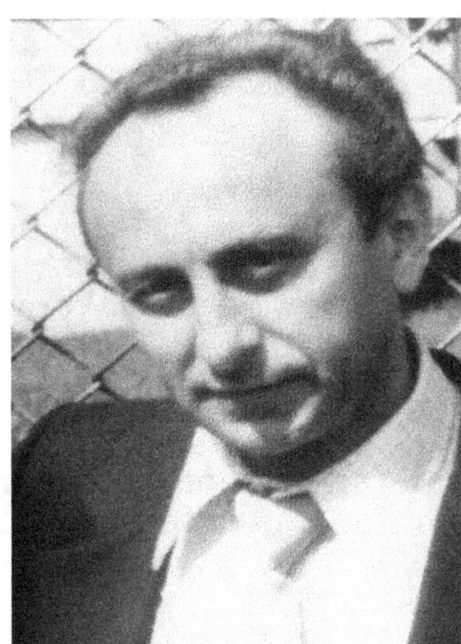

**Fig. 19.** Anton Banko (1927–1986), of Slovenia, who built the first phacoemulsification device as the director of research and development for Cavitron.

to make it suitable for cataract extraction.[70] Navin tasked his engineer, Anton Banko (1927-1986), to develop an ophthalmic prototype. This development took 1 month.[71] Charlie and Banko began working on what they called the "phacoemulsification project" beginning in February 1965, according to Banko's lecture notes.[72] Banko was born in Istria, Croatia (in Yugoslavia), and studied engineering and electronics in Ljubljana, receiving his mechanical engineering degree in 1959. He initially worked in Slovenia as a factory director but then came to the United States with his family, which included two children. They arrived in New York on May 8, 1962. He initially worked as a draftsman, and it was probably in about 1964 when he began working at Cavitron. He had been promoted to the director of research and development before he was tasked to work on the phacoemulsification project (Fig. 19).[73]

It seems that Larry kept up with the project for a while, because Charlie wrote that after several cat experiments had failed, another was attempted, and "Larry was waiting for a call to hear how things had gone."[74]

The original dental Cavitron used nonlongitudinal motion, but this caused iris disinsertion. Charlie wrote: "In 1965, the concept of using a longitudinal motion along the axis of a needle was developed. It was soon noted that high frequency movements were ideal, since no vibrations were visible under the microscope at

---

70 Kelman, 1985, pp. 109-110.

71 Kelman, 1985, pp. 109-110.

72 Allen, 1995. We were provided with these lecture notes by William Banko.

73 Hawlina, 2013, 2014. Interview with William Banko, Jan. 8, 2024.

74 Kelman, 1985, p. 110.

ultrasonic frequencies."[75] Kelman's publications confirm that, at least by 1965, his investigations into the Cavitron for cataract removal were underway.[76]

## Otto Richter (April 1965)

Otto Richter, of Germany, was an instrument maker who began working in the lab between February and April 1965.[77] Kelman explained in a letter to the Hartford Foundation on October 31, 1966, that "Mr. Richter, who works with me at the hospital, is constantly employed in fashioning certain small instruments especially for animal surgery, in maintaining present equipment in the laboratory, and in preparing and developing drills and other equipment unrelated to Cavitron."[78]

## Collaboration with Ronald Odrich (April 1965)

The friendship between Kelman and Odrich involved several new professional and musical collaborations starting in 1965. The first collaboration was professional. Odrich and Kelman discovered that an ophthalmic tool (the cryotherapy probe) could be used for dental procedures. By April 19, 1965, when Kelman wrote his confidential progress report, Kelman had invited Ron Odrich into his lab at the Manhattan Eye Ear, and Throat Hospital as a "visiting dentist"[79]:

> The use of low temperature in Periodental [sic] disease is being investigated in cooperation with Dr. Ronald B. Odrich. It is hoped that this investigation will prove fruitful in correcting deformations such as Gingival pockets, High frenum attachments, interproximal craters, and will facilitate grafting gingiva to correct recession areas.[80]

Odrich had an appointment at Columbia as a periodontist, but he spent every Wednesday working in Kelman's lab. Odrich and Kelman went to Boston to present the periodontal cryotherapy in August 1966, and their work was published in

---

75 Kelman, 1970. A disbursement report covering February 1, 1965, to July 31, 1965 lists $985 for a "probe," while the report covering July 31, 1965, to January 31, 1966, includes $1,491.50 for a "drill" and $1,550 for a "probe," but we are given no further specifics about these instruments (Hartford Foundation files, 1963-1972).

76 Kelman, 1985, p. 121. His July 1967 paper on phacoemulsification was submitted in about October 1966, based on the publication delays noted in his autobiography. In that paper, he indicated that he did 1 year of surgery in cats before working on dogs.

77 Hartford Foundation files, 1963-1972. The progress report of April 1965 noted that Richter was working in the lab part time. Richter first appears in the disbursement report covering February 1 to July 31, 1965.

78 Hartford Foundation files, 1963-1972.

79 Odrich & Kelman, 1967.

80 Hartford Foundation files, 1963-1972.

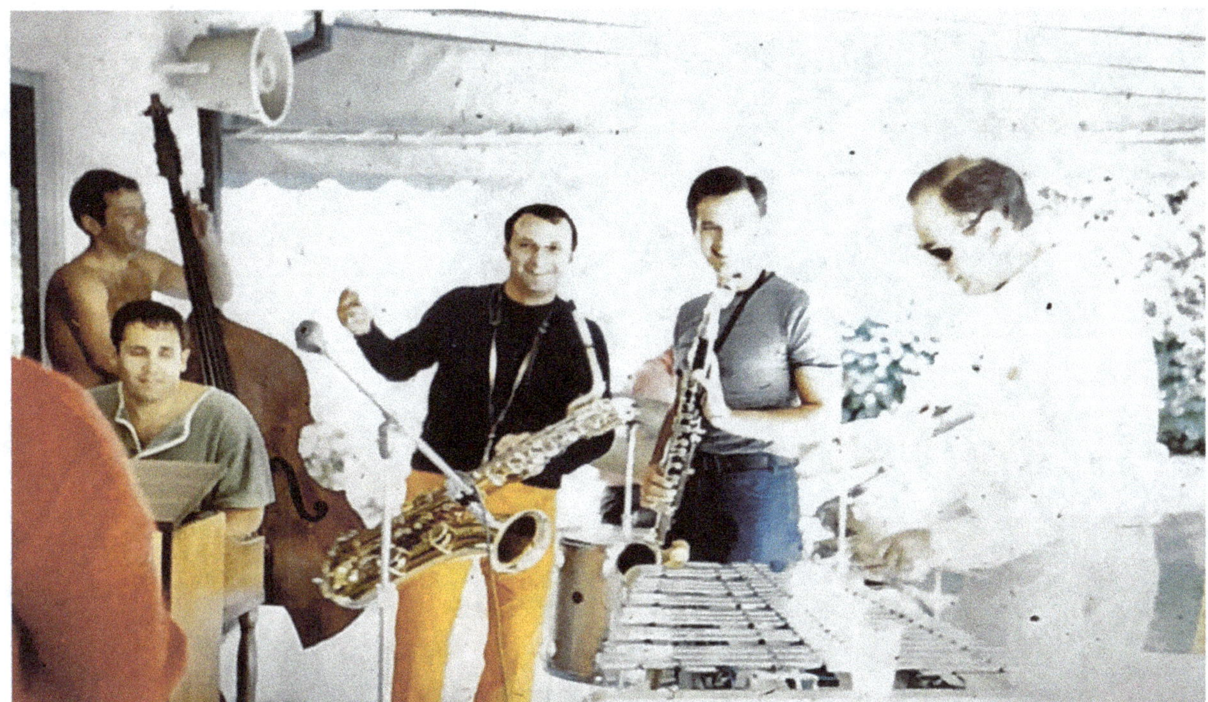

**Fig. 20.** Charlie Kelman with alto saxophone and Ron Odrich with bass clarinet, playing during a party in the backyard near the pool at the Kelman home in Roslyn. Ron estimated this to be in the summer of 1966, close in time to when they went to the Boston cryotherapy conference.

1967.[81] At the lab, Odrich also assisted with anesthesia for cataract surgeries in cats. Kelman told Odrich that he thought he could get Odrich privileges to perform phacoemulsification once the technique was perfected. Odrich found that amusing when he described that to me, but, of course, never pursued it.

Beginning on October 14, 1965, a musician friend of theirs set up weekly Jazz at Noon sessions at New York restaurants, in which musicians with other primary careers (eg, doctors, lawyers, journalists) could improvise together. Ron was involved with Jazz at Noon since its inception in October 1965,[82] and he very quickly convinced Charlie to take time off to participate. Ron, Charlie, and a number of other Jazz at Noon musicians in medicine formed an additional musical group informally known as the Jazz Doctors, which was playing by the late 1960s. Ron would also come by the Kelman home in Roslyn on Sunday afternoons in the late 1960s to play jazz with Charlie (Fig. 20).

---

81 Odrich & Kelman, 1967.

82 *New York Times*, May 25, 1975, pp. 13, 109.

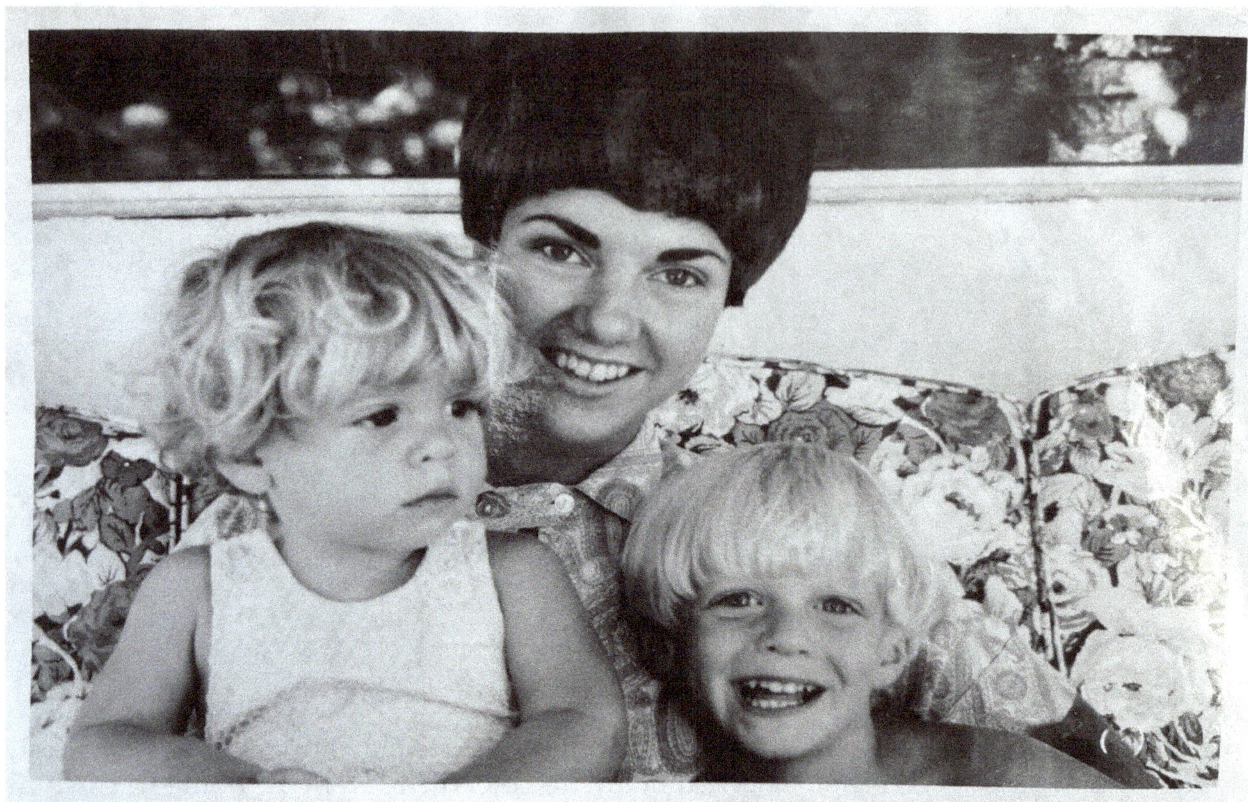

**Fig. 21.** Cheryl Chase (now Jalbert) with Lesley and David Kelman.

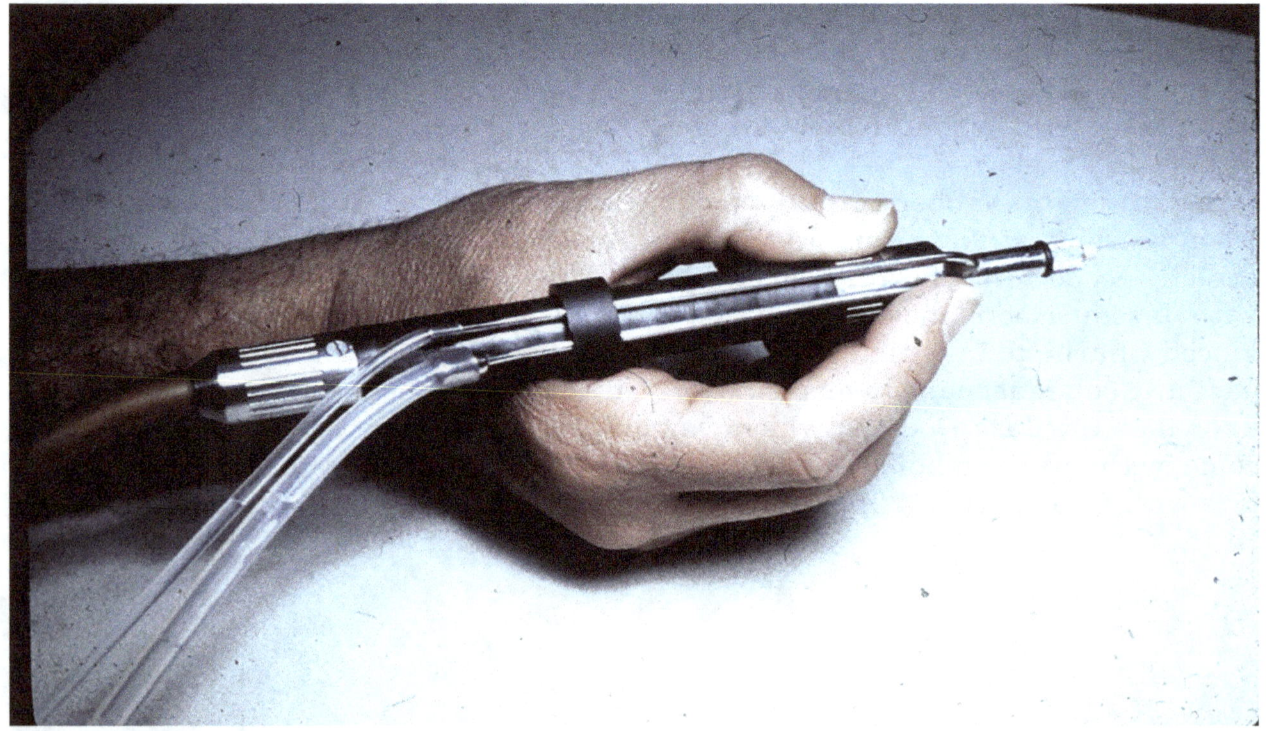

**Fig. 22.** Kelman's hand holding the Kelman phacoemulsification probe in 1971 (Photo courtesy of Norman Medow).

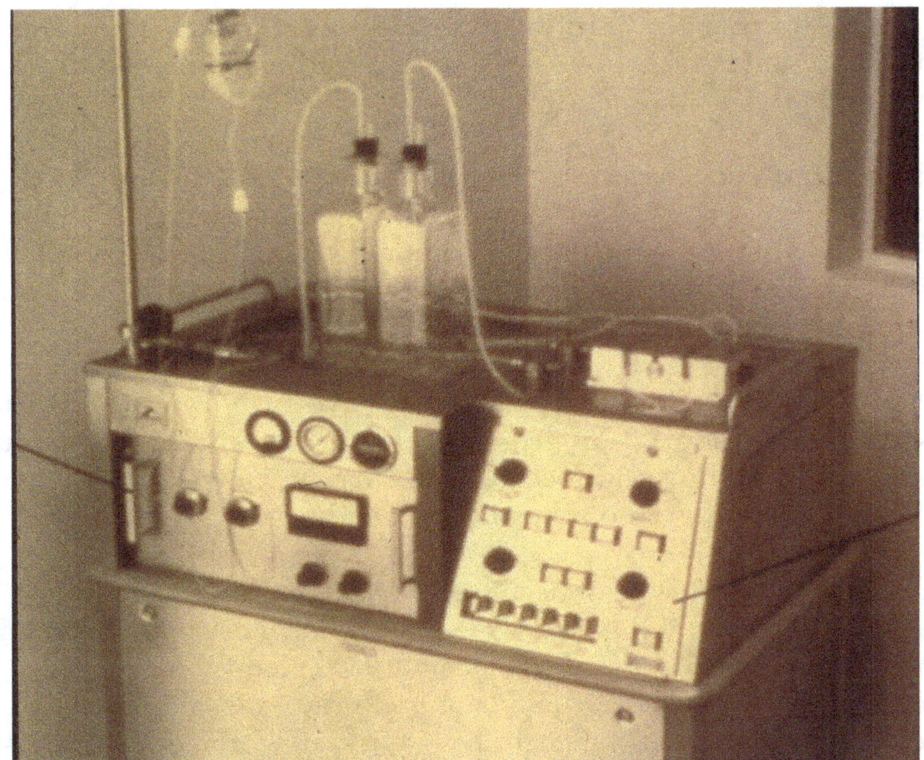

**Fig. 23.** The Kelman phacoemulsifier in 1971 (Photo courtesy of Norman Medow).

## Additional Development of the Phacoemulsification Program (1965)

When Kelman's son David was about 7 months old, in the summer of 1964, Joan hired an 18-year-old girl named Cheryl Chase (now Jalbert) to babysit occasionally (Fig. 21). Cheryl had come to New York from Florida just before her 18th birthday because she wanted to work in the theater, but she ended up working for a textile firm. Joan found Cheryl to be "honest and trustworthy." Joan recommended to Charlie that he hire Cheryl in the lab, which he did in the latter half of 1965.[83] Cheryl remembers that Charlie was still working on cryoextraction of cataracts when she started in the lab, both experimentally and in patients. In addition, Cheryl remembers that when she started working in the lab during the second half of 1965, Charlie was already experimenting with the Cavitron for eye surgery in cats. Cheryl recalled that she started working at the Kelman lab in 1965 before her birthday, which is in September. According to the Foundation reports, Cheryl began working during the August 1, 1965 to Jan. 31, 1966 period, and given that she was paid for the entire six months, it seems that her start date would have been close to August 1, 1965.

---

83 Interview with Cheryl Jalbert, Oct. 2023; Kelman AJO, 1967; Kelman, 1991. Based on the disbursement reports, Cheryl started between August 1, 1965, and January 31, 1966. Cheryl and Joan both remember her starting date as before 1966.

Cheryl remembers that the initial Cavitron handpiece was quite large. Indeed, the first phacoemulsifier handpiece was so heavy that it needed to be suspended above the patient (Figs.s 22 and 23).[84]

Kelman recounted decades later: "By the end of 1965, I had an irrigation and ultrasonic unit that was the forerunner of today's emulsifier."[85] And this landmark was achieved only when he replaced the nonlongitudinal motion, which caused iris disinsertion, with longitudinal motion. In addition, he replaced the stainless steel tip with titanium to prevent flaking.[86]

The first mention of the Cavitron program for eye surgery in the Hartford Foundation files is in a confidential progress report on the small incision surgery program addressed to E. P. Roy and received on April 5, 1966 (Fig. 24). In this report, however, Kelman first described other mechanical attempts:

> A special drill with two micro-surgical blades…was constructed for us by Dr. Martinez and several models of this drill were tried. The blades of this drill rotated in opposite directions and had a 'Waring Blender effect' on the lens. It was possible using these blades to completely emulsify and practically liquify even the most mature cataract. The use of this drill, however, within the eye presents several problems. Because the blades are exposed there was a great tendency for the iris, of the laboratory animals, to become engaged in the blades and destroyed. Several months were spent trying to find a way of protecting the adjacent structures of the eye while maintaining the efficacity of the drills. These drills in combination with a suction device, are being investigated further.

Next, Kelman turned his attention to the Cavitron device:

> In conjunction with Cavitron, Inc., a completely different approach to the destruction of the lens has been devised. A hollow ultrasonic needle was built for us. This needle vibrates at 25,000 cycles per second at a stroke of 5 1/1000 of an inch. When this needle contacts lens substance, it emulsifies the lens and the particles of lens are drawn through the vibrating needle by a gentle suction device. This approach seems to be the most promising at this time. A great deal of time and effort went into the selection of the proper stroke, amplitude and frequency to achieve maximum dissolution of the lens without damaging the adjacent structures. This problem, at this point, seems to be solved. The vibrating tip is protected by a teflon sleeve which avoids a possibility of a corneal burn. Using this instrument, several animals have been successfully operated upon. This, to my knowledge, is the first time that anyone has succeeded in removing a mature lens completely from a living eye through a 1 1/2 or 2 mm opening. These successful cases were performed on March 23, and March 25 of this year 1966. An attempt will now be made to completely refine this

---

84  Kelman, 1991.

85  Kelman, 1994.

86  Kelman, 1994.

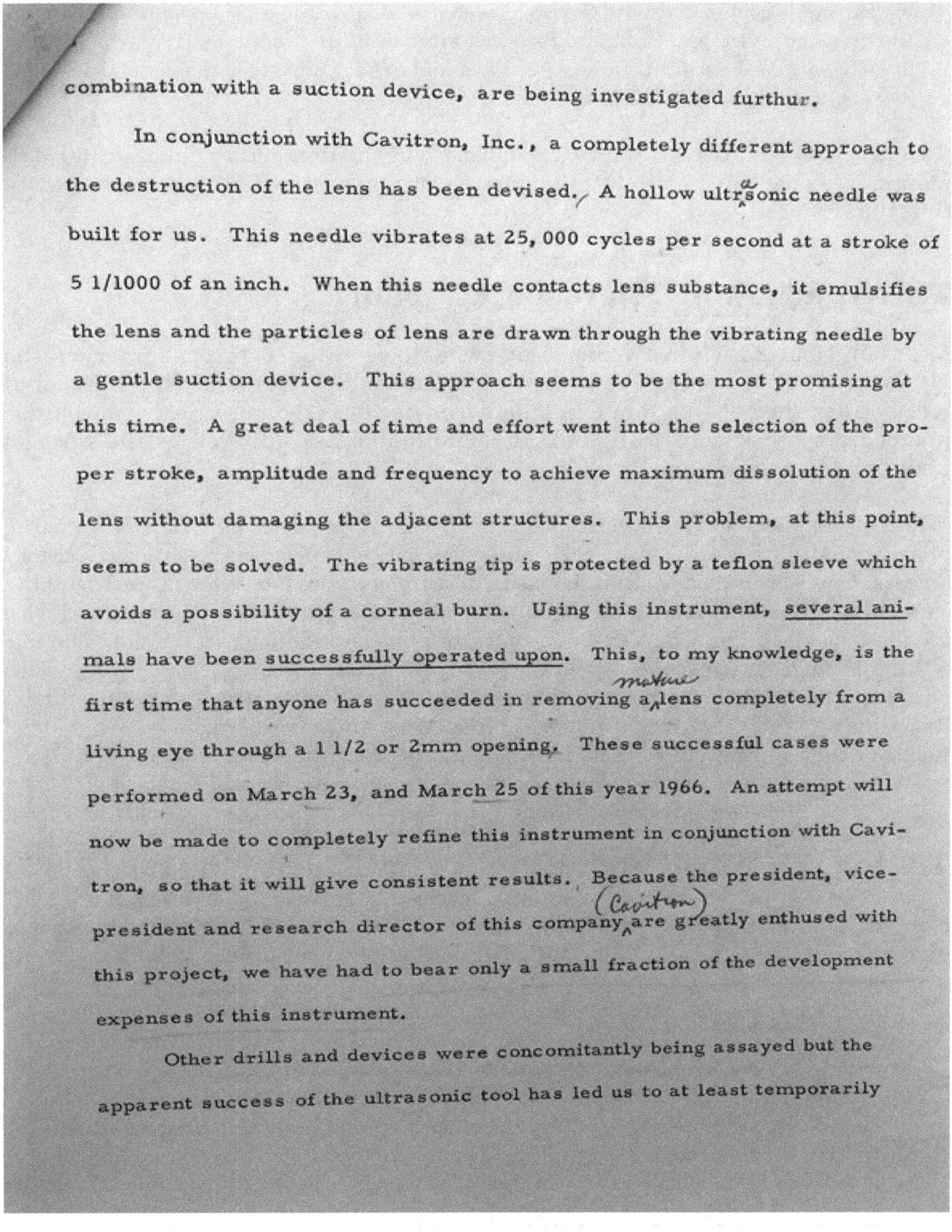

combination with a suction device, are being investigated furthur.

In conjunction with Cavitron, Inc., a completely different approach to the destruction of the lens has been devised. A hollow ultrsonic needle was built for us. This needle vibrates at 25,000 cycles per second at a stroke of 5 1/1000 of an inch. When this needle contacts lens substance, it emulsifies the lens and the particles of lens are drawn through the vibrating needle by a gentle suction device. This approach seems to be the most promising at this time. A great deal of time and effort went into the selection of the proper stroke, amplitude and frequency to achieve maximum dissolution of the lens without damaging the adjacent structures. This problem, at this point, seems to be solved. The vibrating tip is protected by a teflon sleeve which avoids a possibility of a corneal burn. Using this instrument, several animals have been successfully operated upon. This, to my knowledge, is the first time that anyone has succeeded in removing a mature lens completely from a living eye through a 1 1/2 or 2mm opening. These successful cases were performed on March 23, and March 25 of this year 1966. An attempt will now be made to completely refine this instrument in conjunction with Cavitron, so that it will give consistent results. Because the president, vice-president and research director of this company (Cavitron) are greatly enthused with this project, we have had to bear only a small fraction of the development expenses of this instrument.

Other drills and devices were concomitantly being assayed but the apparent success of the ultrasonic tool has led us to at least temporarily

**Fig. 24.** The earliest mention of the Cavitron program in the foundation files in Kelman's confidential progress report addressed to E. P. Roy and received on April 5, 1966 (Hartford Foundation files, 1963–1972).

> instrument in conjunction with Cavitron, so that it will give consistent results. Because the president, vice-president and research director of this company (Cavitron) are greatly enthused with this project, we have had to bear only a small fraction of the development expenses of this instrument.

Note that the March 23, 1966, case in a cat was the first successful case, but Kelman leaves open the possibility that there were unsuccessful cases in cats before that time.

## The Ophthalmic Microscope (1966)

Most surgeons did not use a microscope when performing cataract surgery in the 1960s. In 1966, Richard C. Troutman at Manhattan Eye, Ear, and Throat Hospital received a grant from the Hartford Foundation to advance "stereotactic ophthalmic microsurgery—the substitution of micromanipulators controlled by the surgeon under high magnification."[87]

Ron remembers that Kelman used an operating microscope when performing phacoemulsification even at the early stage when he was performing cataract surgery on cats. Cheryl remembers that despite the secrecy in the lab, some of the residents came in so she could show them the microscope, since it was such an unusual device for the period. Kelman's July 1967 report on phacoemulsification stated: "The use of an operating microscope is mandatory."[88] The press release from the hospital on February 1, 1967, regarding the awarding of the second grant announced that in Kelman's study, "two techniques—cryosurgery and microsurgery—will be used together for the first time."[89] The grant also covered phacoemulsification, but the press release did not mention that technique because it was still a secret.

## Telling the World about Phacoemulsification (1966-1967)

Kelman updated the Hartford Foundation about the status of the Cavitron program on September 30, 1966, when he submitted another grant proposal, which stated:

> ...the fragmenting of cataractous lenses so that they may be withdrawn through a tiny hole in the cornea appears to be the most promising technique. This has been experimentally accomplished by use of a hollow needle vibrating up and down at ultrasonic speed with a stroke of 7/1,000ths of an inch. When the needle is planted in contact with the cataract, the high-frequency motion breaks it down and draws the particles out through the needle by the suction created. This method appears to be feasible as demonstrated by preliminary tests in the laboratory and with the

---

87 Jacobson, 1984, p. 152.

88 Kelman AJO, 1967.

89 Hartford Foundation files, 1963-1972.

human eye...Most of the instruments to be used will be developed in conjunction with Cavitron, Inc., the manufacturers of the ultrasonic equipment.[90]

After his cat work, Kelman had performed experimental phacoemulsification in 30 dogs.[91] The publication indicates that the canine surgeries were performed at the New York Medical College. Indeed, Cheryl remembers them being done at an animal hospital, as well as at the Flower Fifth Avenue Hospital (part of New York Medical College) research department.[92] Cheryl recalled that the first case in dogs was done in the autumn of 1966.

In a progress report received by the Hartford Foundation on April 18, 1967, Kelman reported that in the past year (Fig. 25):

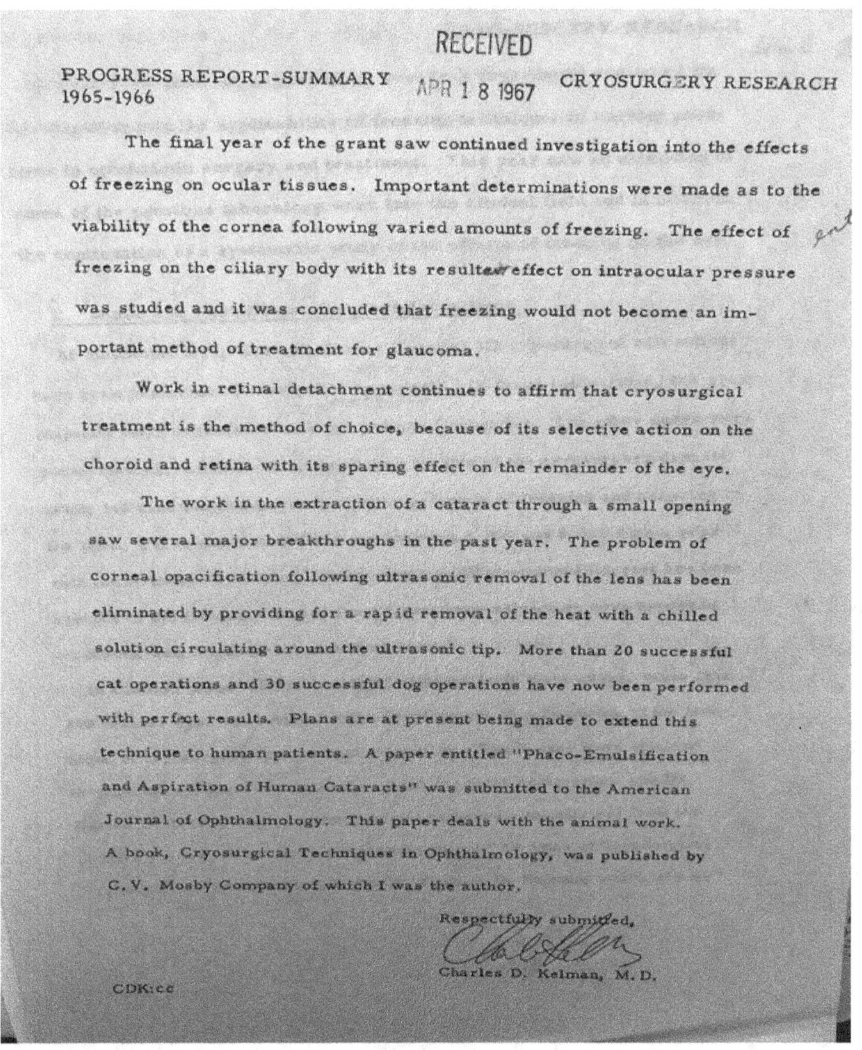

RECEIVED

PROGRESS REPORT-SUMMARY          APR 1 8 1967          CRYOSURGERY RESEARCH
1965-1966

The final year of the grant saw continued investigation into the effects of freezing on ocular tissues. Important determinations were made as to the viability of the cornea following varied amounts of freezing. The effect of freezing on the ciliary body with its resultant effect on intraocular pressure was studied and it was concluded that freezing would not become an important method of treatment for glaucoma.

Work in retinal detachment continues to affirm that cryosurgical treatment is the method of choice, because of its selective action on the choroid and retina with its sparing effect on the remainder of the eye.

The work in the extraction of a cataract through a small opening saw several major breakthroughs in the past year. The problem of corneal opacification following ultrasonic removal of the lens has been eliminated by providing for a rapid removal of the heat with a chilled solution circulating around the ultrasonic tip. More than 20 successful cat operations and 30 successful dog operations have now been performed with perfect results. Plans are at present being made to extend this technique to human patients. A paper entitled "Phaco-Emulsification and Aspiration of Human Cataracts" was submitted to the American Journal of Ophthalmology. This paper deals with the animal work. A book, Cryosurgical Techniques in Ophthalmology, was published by C. V. Mosby Company of which I was the author.

Respectfully submitted,

Charles D. Kelman, M.D.

CDK:cc

**Fig. 25.** Kelman's progress report describing phacoemulsification in cats and dogs, received by the Hartford Foundation on April 18, 1967.

---

90  Hartford Foundation files, 1963-1972.

91  Kelman AJO, 1967.

92  Kelman AJO, 1967.

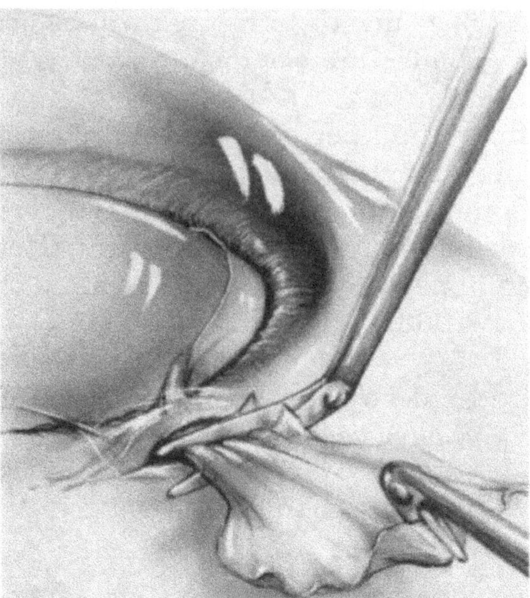

**Fig. 26.** The base of the anterior capsule was cut with the capsule external to the eye (Kelman AJO 1967).

> The problem of corneal opacification following ultrasonic removal of the lens has been eliminated by providing for a rapid removal of the heat with a chilled solution circulating around the ultrasonic tip. More than 20 successful cat operations and 30 successful dog operations have now been performed with perfect results. Plans are at present being made to extend this technique to human patients.

Kelman also indicated that his first paper on the topic had been submitted. In this July 1967 report, Kelman described his experiences with phacoemulsification to remove the crystalline lens in "more than 200 cadavers, 40 cats and 30 dogs" in July 1967.[93] Kelman later wrote that this article was accepted several weeks after submission and that it appeared in print "about nine months" later.[94] Therefore, Kelman probably submitted the paper in the latter half of 1966. He explained that he had been working on some type of enzymatic or mechanical means of liquefying cataracts for 4 years. He had performed most of the work at the Cryo-Research Department of the Manhattan Eye, Ear, and Throat Hospital. The work was funded from a grant from the John A. Hartford Foundation. His goal was to enable aspiration of a mature cataract through a 2- to 3-mm incision. Kelman explained that enzymatic means to dissolve cataracts would probably damage other intraocular structures.

The ultrasonic transducer and the suction were controlled by independent foot switches. He dilated the pupil preoperatively with subconjunctival Cyclogyl and adrenaline. He began the procedure with a large air bubble in the anterior chamber.

---

93  Kelman AJO, 1967.
94  Kelman, 1985, p. 121.

A V-shaped capsulorrhexis was performed, and the V-shaped portion of the anterior capsule was withdrawn from the eye, with an assistant cutting the base of the V-shaped capsule outside the eye (Fig. 26).

A small metal lens loop was inserted into the crystalline lens, posterior to its nucleus, and moved anteriorly to sublux the nucleus into the anterior chamber. The lens loop was then withdrawn from the eye, and phacoemulsification of the nucleus and much of the cortex was performed. Then, residual lens cortex was aspirated (Fig. 27).

In animals, Kelman left the posterior capsule, because it was attached to the anterior hyaloid face, and its removal would cause vitreous loss. Kelman placed a corneal suture and also sutured animal lids closed. In human (cadaver) eyes, Kelman used a 3-minute application of alpha-chymotrypsin to dissolve the zonules and then grasped the anterior capsule, removing it from the eye and bringing with it the posterior capsule. Thus, this preliminary report concerned intracapsular cataract extraction. (The entire lens capsule was removed.) Kelman indicated that there were fewer complications in the cats as he gained more experience, and the final four cats had no complications. Some of the early cats experienced complete corneal opacification, which Kelman attributed to excessive heat, lenticular contact with the corneal endothelium, and other factors. If the posterior capsule was ruptured, Kelman extended the incision to 180° (6 o'clock hours) and extracted the lens with the cryoextractor. Kelman was able to reduce the degree of fibrinous exudate in the anterior chamber postoperatively using heparin in the irrigating solution. Kelman did not experiment on dog eyes until he had 1 year experience with cats. He also operated successfully on several dogs with cataracts (as opposed to experimental clear lensectomies). Kelman applied phacoemulsification in vitro to "approximately 300 cataractous lenses removed by conventional techniques in surgery."[95] Kelman experimented on cadaver eyes, which had edematous corneas. He, therefore, removed the cornea and iris before surgical experiments.

Cheryl was consistent in reporting that the first human case was in April 1967. The night before this surgery, she slept in the nurse's locker room with the phacoemulsification unit, because she did not want anyone to find out what they were doing, or to disturb the machine. In an addendum to the July 1967 report, Kelman explained that he had performed removal of cataracts by phacoemulsification in two volunteers with blind eyes, to demonstrate the feasibility of the technique.[96] Cheryl remembers that Banko was present at the first phacoemulsification in a human 1967, and for subsequent surgeries in humans. Banko's son indicated that it was important to have an engineer present for critical surgeries, as in humans, because the early phacoemulsifiers had to be properly tuned to find the resonant frequency for the nickel transducer.

---

95 Kelman AJO, 1967.
96 Kelman AJO, 1967.

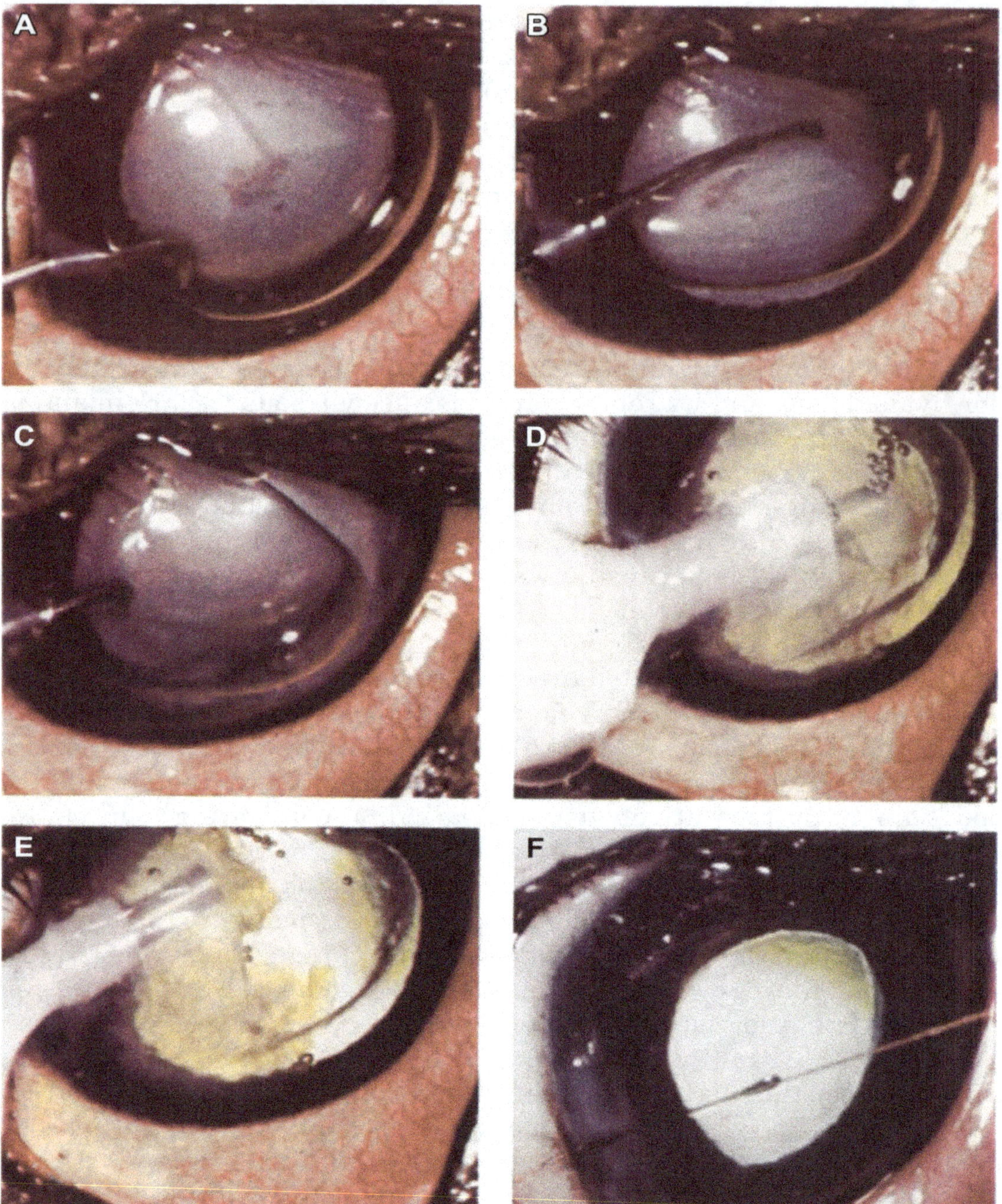

**Fig. 27.** "A. A cystotome enters anterior chamber through a 2-mm shelved incision. Air fills anterior chamber. Pupil is well dilated. B. The cystotome engages capsule of lens at a point opposite the incision. C. A V-shaped opening made in capsule. The cystotome withdraws capsule from the chamber and the capsule is cut (not shown). D. Phacoemulsifier introduced into lens mass. Irrigation, sonic-ultrasonic energy, and aspiration are employed. E. Sharp edges of lens material demonstrate solid nature of cataract. Teflon sleeve protects cornea. Lens half removed in 4 minutes. F. Lens completely removed, except for posterior capsule, in 6 minutes. One suture placed." (Kelman AJO 1967).

On July 25, 1967, the Cavitron Corporation filed a patent entitled "Material removal apparatus and method employing high frequency vibrations," with the inventors listed as Charles Kelman and Anton Banko. As the patent was not granted until 1971, it expired in 1988.

Kelman presented his paper to the Manhattan Eye, Ear, and Throat Hospital on July 27, 1967. C. G. Coggins of the Hartford Foundation sat in on the proceedings and filed a memorandum about it. Kelman showed a "sound-color film of 7 minutes" on phacoemulsification. Regarding John McClean of Cornell, Coggins wrote:

> His questions were piercing and at first apparently antagonistic but he ended up with a statement to the effect that the technique, if developed, could be a great contribution and was highly ingenious.[97]

## The Second Grant Period (1967–1968)

Kelman's grant was due to expire at the start of 1967. Kelman explained some of the proposed costs in a letter to the Hartford Foundation on October 31, 1966:

> The other funds for instrument development [in the grant] are to be used to pay for engineering and research done for us with companies such as Cavitron. At this time, Cavitron has already spent more than ten thousand dollars directly related to our project, for which they have not expected reimbursement. In the future, however, they will probably expect reimbursement for their efforts until such a time as the operation becomes feasible and practical...It has very recently become apparent that twenty-five thousand cycles at a stroke of 7/1000 of an inch has some tardive effects on the corneal endothelium and it will be necessary to construct other equipment which will function at a lower cycle. The figure of ten thousand dollars for instrument development in the first and second years is a realistic one.[98]

Kelman was presumably satisfied with the progress made in 1968 (Figure 28). He used the code "1968" for years for keypad entry into buildings.[99] The progress report to the Hartford Foundation from March 8, 1968, showed how much smaller the phacoemulsification handpiece had become.

In April 1969, Kelman detailed the technique and outcome of phacoemulsification in 12 human patients.[100] He explained that his goal was to eliminate the need for "hospitalization and convalescence," using a 2-mm limbal incision, which required only one absorbable suture for the primary incision.[101] He actually made an incision

---

97 Hartford Foundation files, 1963-1972.

98 Hartford Foundation files, 1963-1972.

99 Interview with Lesley Koeppel, October 2023.

100 Kelman AJO, 1969.

101 Kelman AJO, 1969.

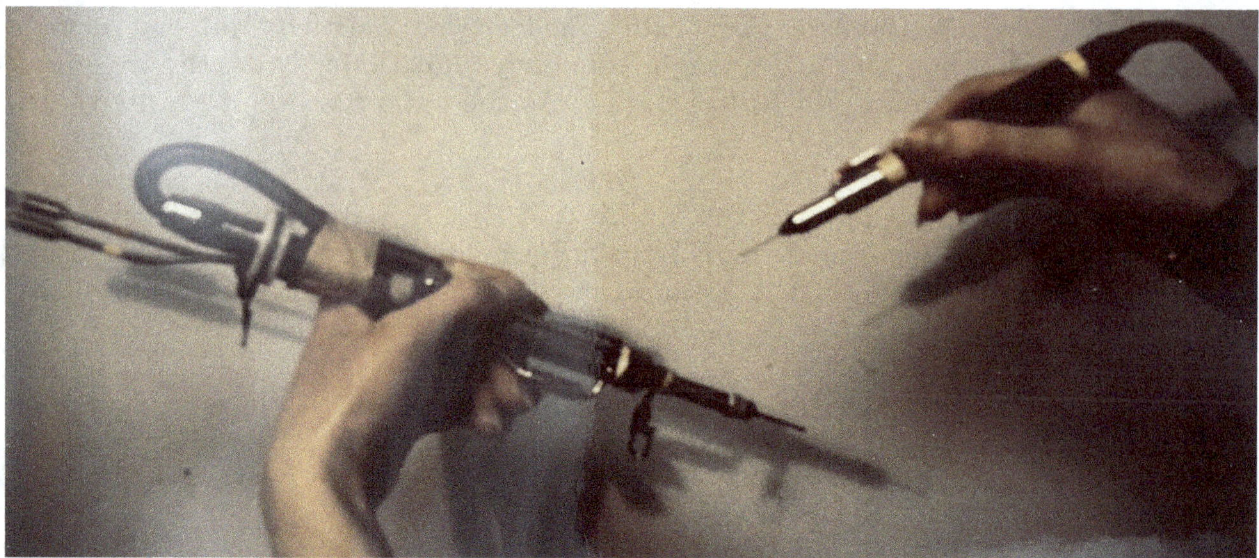

**Fig. 28.** Decrease in the size of the phacoemulsification from the original (left) and by March 8, 1968 (Hartford Foundation files 1963-1972).

through the conjunctiva just superior to the superior limbus to create a flap, before incising the corneoscleral limbus. Most of his patients were older and had "hard, mature lenses." Eight of the 12 patients had retinal disease. He dilated the pupils with atropine, Cyclogyl, and Neo-Synephrine eye drops, reserving subconjunctival Cyclogyl injections for persistent poor dilation. A Zeiss operating microscope with magnification of 6× to 10× was used. He performed V-shaped anterior capsulotomy as before. He again prolapsed the lens into the anterior chamber to perform phacoemulsification there, but did not depict using a lens loop. He again placed alpha-chymotrypsin behind the iris to dissolve the zonules and removed the anterior capsule and the attached posterior capsule. In addition to the single suture for the limbal incision, three absorbable sutures were placed in the conjunctiva. Kelman noted that "the patient immediately is allowed unrestricted activity." In addition, a contact lens could be worn "almost immediately." In addition to atropine drops and Maxitrol, he prescribed Diamox 250 mg twice daily for 3 days. He often left the eye unpatched after surgery. He described a "striate keratitis" caused by corneal edema and Descemet folds. He lost vitreous in 2 of the 12 cases.

In an addendum, Kelman explained that since manuscript preparation, more than 40 additional cases of cataract phacoemulsification had been performed.[102] He noted four cases of "eight-ball hemorrhage" causing glaucoma, treated by emulsification and aspiration of the blood through a corneal incision. He had also used this technique for traumatic and congenital cataracts and for a dislocated lens in patient with Marfan.

---

102  Kelman AJO, 1969.

By May 1973, Kelman had performed 800 cases of phacoemulsification, and about 3,500 cases had been performed nationwide.[103] Kelman regarded brunescent cataracts as a contraindication in the older patients. By 1973, Kelman typically left the posterior capsule in place and was, therefore, performing extracapsular extraction, although if he doubted the posterior capsule clarity, he made a small central posterior capsulotomy, while endeavoring to leave the vitreous face intact. In the first 500 cases, "aphakic glaucoma" occurred in only one case, possibly because the vitreous adhered to the cornea. Posterior capsular rupture occurred in 9% of cases. When vitreous was lost, Kelman injected air into the anterior chamber and swept the wound. Vitreous loss caused peaked pupils postoperatively in 7% of the first 100 patients, but this rate was subsequently reduced to 1%. Five of 500 patients had retinal detachments postoperatively. Two patients had the "Irvine-Gass syndrome" (macular edema), one of whom had leakage of fluorescein in the macula. Two patients suffered "complete loss of vision," which was attributed to the retrobulbar injection of lidocaine in one case and a central retinal artery occlusion from massage in the other case.

## Intraocular Lenses (1968)

Kelman recognized that placing a standard intraocular lens in the eye would require enlargement of the incision after phacoemulsification, and so he sought to create an intraocular lens compatible with small incision surgery. In his third grant proposal, submitted to the Hartford Foundation on July 26, 1968, Kelman proposed what he called "Phaco-Replacement with an Artificial Intraocular Lens." (Fig. 29)

Kelman wrote in the proposal:

> It is our aim to introduce into the small incision required for Phaco-Emulsification an expandable silicon membrane into which silicon fluid or other plastic would be introduced and sealed. It might be possible to, thereby, introduce into the eye a lens which would exactly match the patient's need for glasses, following cataract surgery.[104]

Kelman's progress report, which the Foundation received on March 30, 1970, stated:

> Work on the intra ocular plastic lens has not passed the preliminary stage. It has recently been learned that even the 'inert' plastics cause some reaction after several years. A special glass lens may prove inert, but we are awaiting the results of other's research on the matter.[105]

Ultimately, some years later, Kelman produced a lens with haptics, resembling a triangle missing one side. This lens was known as a "pregnant 7" due to its appearance.

---

103  Kelman AJO, 1973.
104  Hartford Foundation files, 1963-1972.
105  Hartford Foundation files, 1963-1972.

52

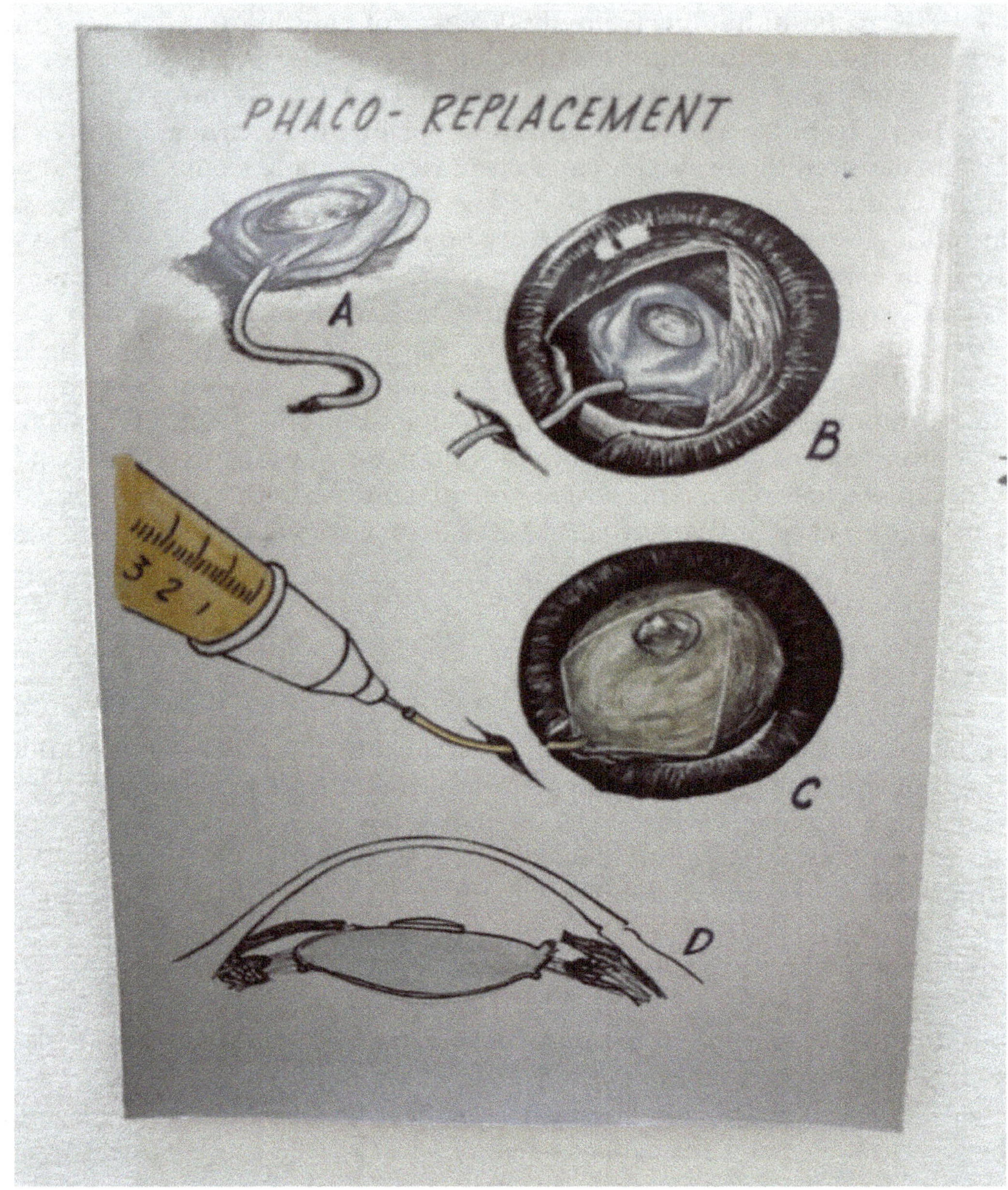



**Fig. 29.** Phaco-replacement from Kelman grant proposal of July 26, 1968.

## Pure Carbon in Ophthalmology (1972).

In 1972, Kelman applied for further funding from the Hartford Foundation, with a grant entitled: "Investigation of Applications of Pure Carbon in Ophthalmology." Kelman noted that pure carbon elicited no fibroplastic or foreign body reaction. He sought to use pure carbon to develop "1) corneal prosthetics, 2) glaucoma setons, and 3) intraocular retinal pins." He also proposed using a diamond intraocular lens after cataract surgery, and a carbon "ball" as a prosthesis after enucleation. He reviewed the use of carbon in cardiology. This grant received negative evaluations by two consultants, including A. Edward Maumenee of Wilmer. The consultants mentioned not only the scientific merit, but also the publicity which attended Kelman's use of phacoemulsification, which they seemed to view in a negative light. The Foundation did not fund this proposal, citing both the scientific evaluations, the duration of prior funding, and other issues of a "general" nature. The Foundation indicated that he could fund his research through his own educational foundation. Kelman never applied for funding from the Foundation again.

## Business Considerations (1971–1978)

In 1971, the Hartford Foundation files depict a crisis for Kelman. The Public Broadcasting Service (PBS) documentary from 2010 indicated that Kelman had a business arrangement with Cavitron. Someone complained to the Foundation that Kelman was profiting inappropriately from the cryotherapy and phacoemulsification devices. In a letter to the Hartford Foundation dated October 4, 1971, Kelman wrote he believed the complainant was a doctor at his hospital. Kelman's letter stated: "Because of the research funds given by the John A. Hartford Foundation, and because my father, David J. Kelman, left me sufficient personal funds to live comfortably, I have been able to devote the past eight years to helping others, using the inventive aptitudes which he also passed on to me."[106] Kelman also wrote on October 4, 1971, that "the implication that I received royalties on freezing, ultrasonic or any other devices is entirely untrue" and that "the unregistered warrants given by Frigitronics were in no way a royalty—merely an unsolicited charitable gift [to Kelman's educational foundation]. The warrants were never executed, and their exact value is questionable and probably not very great at this time."[107] A telegram from Ralph E. Crump, the president of Frigitronics, on October 2, 1971, to the Foundation stated that Crump had known Kelman since early 1963 when they began producing a cataract and then a retinal cryoprobe and that Kelman refused royalties, but that "in the early 1970 [sic] when all of his cryo researched [sic] was behind him, myself and one other principal made a rather small peronnel [sic] donation to his research fund of warrants for unregistered stock…"[108] A telegram from Navin, the president of Cavitronics, to

---

106  Hartford Foundation files, 1963-1972.

107  Hartford Foundation files, 1963-1972.

108  Hartford Foundation files, 1963-1972.

the Foundation on October 4, 1971, stated: "Dr. Kelman has devoted extensively of his energies and talents to this promising procedure and we are grateful to him for what has been accomplished. Cavitron has not paid Kelman any royalties directly or indirectly as a result of this effort. Should Cavitron's program become commercially successful Cavitron would expect to help Kelman's teaching programs in ways felt to be appropriate to the purpose."[109]

A related crisis came later in the 1970s. Cavitron became mired in legal disputes with several companies who sought to manufacture phacoemulsification devices. Anton Banko had to provide sworn testimony for depositions with regard to the Cavitron patents.[110]

On February 11, 1975, Coburn of the Hartford Foundation wrote a memo indicating that he had spoken with an attorney named J. Ralph King who represented Calusonics of California, a company working on a phacoemulsification device. King wanted to know "...whether they need a licence to go ahead and whether the patent holders could be compelled to give it in view of Foundation financing." Coburn recorded that "there is nothing and to my knowledge there never has been anything on the patenting and licencing of the device. We were just never advised in writing."[111] Coburn wrote to King the same day about the relevant grant language: "No person, firm or corporation...shall have any proprietary interest of whatever nature in any results or ideas developed or established in the prosecution of the project to be underwritten hereby...Our files do not indicate that any exceptions were made."[112]

Note that Coburn indicated that the Foundation was never "advised in writing." This leaves open the possibility that Kelman did discuss it verbally with someone at the Foundation. Indeed, there is a cryptic handwritten note in the Foundation files, with the date "7/24/67" on the top line (Fig. 30). That is the day before the patent was filed. This handwritten note refers to a patent by Kelman and Cavitron and reads "no restriction" and notes that "we [apparently the Foundation] are not party to Agreement." Perhaps, Kelman had informal discussions with someone at the Foundation about the patent before it was filed and thought he had received permission.

On July 28, 1975, Kelman wrote a letter to Robert E. Navin of the Cavitron Corporation (Fig. 31A,B): "The first grant that I received from the Hartford Foundation was in 1963, and this grant was for the development of cryo-surgical techniques in ophthalmology. There was no application for or use of funds for developing a phaco-emulsifier instrument."[113] Kelman continued that on the second grant, which he dated to 1966, "The objective of this research is to perfect the *technique* which has already been discovered by this investigator...The above two quotes clearly

---

109  Hartford Foundation files, 1963-1972.
110  William Banko, personal communication, January 8, 2024.
111  Hartford Foundation files, 1963-1972.
112  Hartford Foundation files, 1963-1972.
113  Hartford Foundation files, 1963-1972.

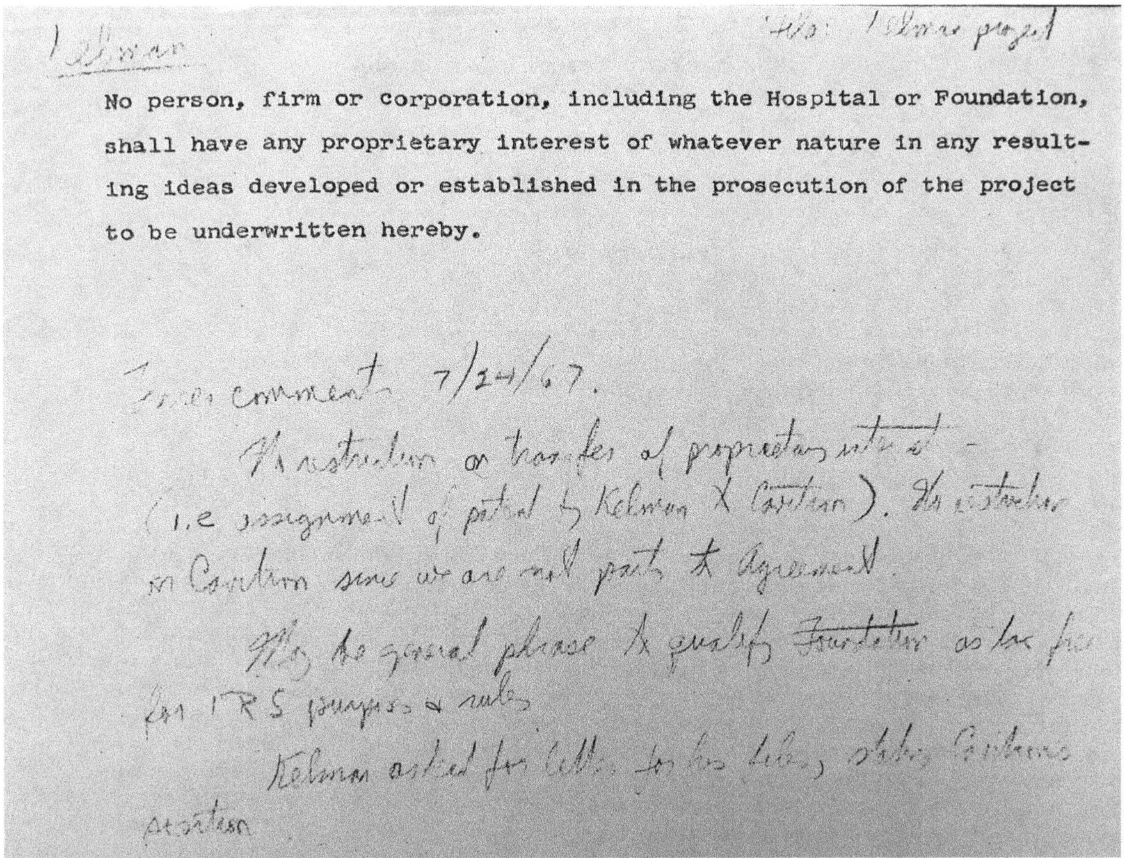

**Fig. 30.** Handwritten note in the Hartford Foundation files, which seems to suggest that the Foundation might have been aware of the agreement between Kelman and Cavitron regarding the phacoemulsification patent on July 24, 1967, the day before the patent was filed.

indicate the Hartford Foundation Grant was given to develop the technique, and that the instrument to be finally designed would be left to Cavitron...Since the Hartford Foundation funds did not support the development of the phaco-emulsifier as an instrument, but only supported the work in the laboratory involving animal experiments and clinical evaluation later on, there is obviously no conflict of interest. Unless it could be shown (which of course it cannot) that the Cavitron/Kelman Phaco-Emulsifier was developed with research funds from the Hartford Foundation, the allegations in Mr. King's letter are entirely off base."[114]

A profile from July 25, 1976, stated that the idea to use the Cavitron for cataract surgery occurred to Kelman "with $255,000 of the funding and all but three months of the research time spent."[115] The reporter who interviewed Kelman also indicated that he had a "new (and uncharacteristic) reluctance" to talk about his medical research.[116]

---

114 Hartford Foundation files, 1963-1972.

115 Lowe, 1976, pp. 7-10.

116 Lowe, 1976, pp. 7-10.

CHARLES D. KELMAN, M. D.
150 EAST 58th STREET
NEW YORK, N. Y. 10022

PLaza 2-8030

July 28, 1975

Mr. Robert E. Navin
1290 Avenue of the Americas
26th Floor
New York, New York

Dear Mr. Navin:

Thank you for your letter of July 7th with the enclosure from Mr. Ralph King. The implications and conclusions of Mr. King's letter are entirely erroneous and I have looked into the matter both with Mr. Coburn and Mr. Long. The facts are as follows. The first grant that I received from the Hartford Foundation was in 1963, and this grant was for the development of cryo-surgical techniques in ophthalmology. There was no application for or use of funds for developing a phaco-emulsifier instrument. This grant lasted three years and was subsequently renewed. The second grant from the Hartford Foundation was given in 1966 and the title of the grant was Cryo-Surgery and Other Investigative Surgery in Ophthalmology. That grant application was for the continuation of investigation of cryo-surgery and other investigative surgery in ophthalmology. Under this category would fall the designation of investigation of the technique of small incision cataract surgery. I quote from page three of this grant application. "The objective of this research is to perfect the technique which has already been discovered by this investigator." Further along in the same grant application, and again I quote 'most of the instruments to be used will be developed in conjunction with Cavitron Corporation the manufacturers of the ultra-sonic equipment. Other instruments will be developed for ancillary procedures with whatever surgical company is best suited. "

The above two quotes clearly indicate the Hartford Foundation Grant was given to develop the technique, and that the instrument to be finally designed would be left to Cavitron. This was stated in the grant and accepted as such. Since the Hartford Foundation funds did not support the development of the phaco-emulsifier as an instrument, but only supported the work in the laboratory involving animal experiments and clinical evaluation later on, there is obviously no conflict of interest.

Unless it could be shown (which of course it cannot) that the Cavitron/Kelman Phaco-Emulsifier was developed with research funds from the Hartford Foundation, the allegations in Mr. King's letter are entirely off base.

A

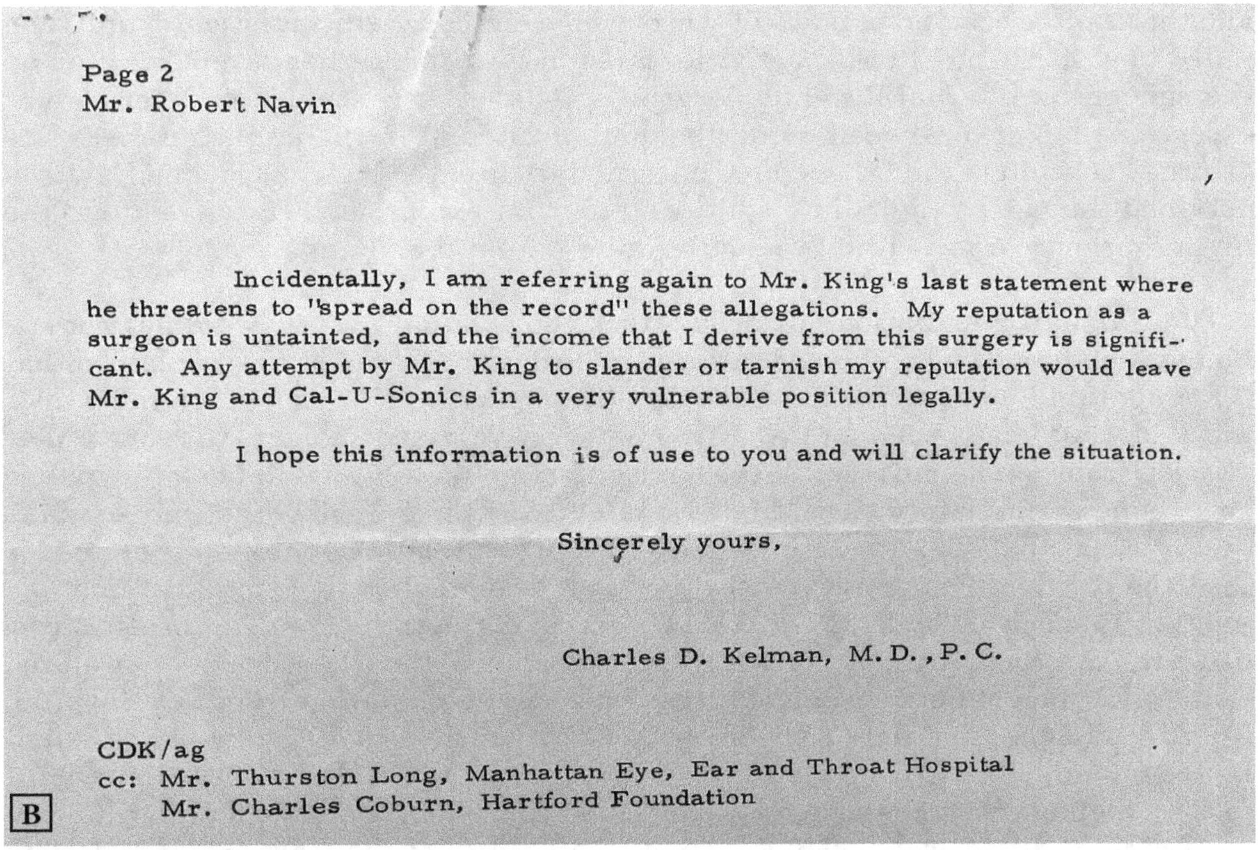

Page 2
Mr. Robert Navin

Incidentally, I am referring again to Mr. King's last statement where he threatens to "spread on the record" these allegations. My reputation as a surgeon is untainted, and the income that I derive from this surgery is significant. Any attempt by Mr. King to slander or tarnish my reputation would leave Mr. King and Cal-U-Sonics in a very vulnerable position legally.

I hope this information is of use to you and will clarify the situation.

Sincerely yours,

Charles D. Kelman, M.D., P.C.

CDK/ag
cc: Mr. Thurston Long, Manhattan Eye, Ear and Throat Hospital
    Mr. Charles Coburn, Hartford Foundation

**B**

**Fig. 31A-B.** On July 28, 1978, Kelman wrote that the development of the phacoemulsification device did not use funding from a nonprofit organization (the Hartford Foundation), and therefore, by implication, the patent was valid.

The patent disputes continued. On August 18, 1977, an attorney for Fibra-Sonics, Inc. of Chicago indicated that the company had been sued by Cavitron. The attorney stated that they believed Hartford Foundation funds had been used to develop phacoemulsification, and they further noted that "...inventions conceived or first reduced to practice under grants from the John A. Hartford Foundation would be dedicated to the good of all mankind in that a patent rights clause would be included in such grants."[117] On September 23, 1977, the Hartford Foundation attorneys wrote to Kelman that they had spoken with the hospital attorneys about the Fibra-Sonics/Cavitron dispute and stated: "We are left with an unclear picture as to your relationship to Cavitron...the Internal Revenue Code that prohibits the use of charitable funds to benefit a private interest. In the context of the Foundation's medical research grants, this admonition is meant to prevent the situation where an investigator develops a process through charitable funding, patents it in his own name and then exploits it for commercial purposes. As you can imagine, where something along these lines occurs the organization which made the grant

---

117 Hartford Foundation files, 1963-1972.

and the grantee hospital or medical school which employed the investigator and then failed to properly monitor his activities must face up to a rather severe reaction on the part of the Internal Revenue Service."[118] The letter continued to describe how exceptions might have been requested, and granted, if in the public interest. The attorney continued that "...we are concerned to discover by what means Cavitron obtained the patent rights in dispute and to what extent such rights relate to the investigations carried out by you with funding from the Foundation."[119]

The Hartford Foundation's attorneys took the position that they did not know if Foundation funds had been used to develop the device. The attorneys explained that if Foundation funds had been used to develop phacoemulsification, then the proper protocol would have been for any of the prospective patent holders to request permission from the Foundation. If the device were going to be available to the public on a "nondiscriminatory basis" and if a patent was the only practical way to make the device available to the public, then an exemption could be granted. But, in this case, the Hartford Foundation determined that no one asked them for an exemption. A letter from November 21, 1978, from De Forest & Duer, the Foundation attorneys, listed the contract language and the relevant section of the IRS code and then stated that "...we have no knowledge of a request to the Foundation from the Hospital, from Dr. Kelman or from Cavitron, Inc,—with which corporation we understand Dr. Kelman is affiliated—for a release or waiver of any rights reserved pursuant to the language recited above."[120] After 1978, E. P. Roy, the key administrator on the Kelman grants, was no longer listed as an officer of the Hartford Foundation, ending 27 years of service.[121]

## Hypotheses Regarding the Timeline.

It is strange that the development of phacoemulsification should be such a landmark in the history of ophthalmology, but that so little should have been known about the specifics of the timeline. It seems logical that the secrecy surrounding the project should have kept the ophthalmic community in the dark at the time, but why wouldn't the timeline be made public when the device was revealed to the world in 1967? Why didn't Kelman make specific statements about the dates when he first learned of the Cavitron, first saw the Cavitron, first tested it in an eye, and first initiated his formal Cavitron research program? If these events really had all occurred on the same day, as stipulated in his autobiography, wouldn't he want to tell us the date, or at least the year? Why did Charlie continue the secrecy long after the world knew about the device? We evaluated several hypotheses, which are not mutually exclusive, and could have all contributed.

---

118  Hartford Foundation files, 1963-1972.

119  Hartford Foundation files, 1963-1972.

120  Hartford Foundation files, 1963-1972.

121  Jacobson, 1984, p. 247.

One hypothesis we considered relates to Charlie's skill as a raconteur and entertainer. The story that he told of proceeding through all the steps from serendipitously learning of the Cavitron's existence while having his teeth cleaned, running out of the dental office with exclamations of joy, testing the Cavitron on a cataract successfully, and initiating a formal research program, all on the same day, within a few months of the grant expiring, is a wonderful modern retelling of the eureka moment of Archimedes in the bath. In the PBS documentary, Charlie actually called it his "eureka" moment. In his autobiography, Charlie added the comedic element that he seemed so crazy when he returned to Larry's office that the dentist held up a needle as if to sedate Charlie to calm him down. It is a story that has resonated with generations of ophthalmologists and laypeople. His autobiography became a best-seller. Kelman told the newspapers that he hoped his story would be turned into a musical, and later that it would be turned into a TV movie. The latter did ultimately happen, in 2010, when a documentary was made about his life.

Our perusal of the Hartford Foundation files brought to light another hypothesis: preservation of the Kelman/Banko/Cavitron patent. If Kelman stumbled upon the Cavitron dental instrument towards the very end of the grant period, and it turned out it just happened to work for eye surgery too with minimal modification, it would be easier to claim that funds from the Hartford Foundation, a tax-exempt nonprofit organization, were not used to develop phacoemulsification. It would be easier for Kelman to claim that he was just a product tester, and surgical technique innovator, rather than a medical device inventor (Kelman 1994).

## Hypotheses Regarding the Involvement of Dentists.

In addition to the timeline, another mystery concerns the involvement of two dentists, when Charlie always told the story as involving just one dentist. By every account from Charlie's public writings and statements, and the public and private statements of Larry, both Charlie and Larry were together: when Charlie first saw the Cavitron, when Larry explained to Charlie how it worked by acceleration, when the idea was formulated to use the Cavitron for cataract surgery, and when the first test of the Cavitron on a crystalline lens was performed at Larry's office. Moreover, Charlie wrote that he kept Larry apprised of the early results in cats. Thus, all of these accounts are consistent with the concept that the earliest phacoemulsification work was a collaboration between Charlie and Larry, his dentist. According to his son, Larry was "gentle". Joan recalled Larry's generosity in being willing to accede to her request for a higher salary when she worked for him. Larry never publicly sought any more credit in the early development of phacoemulsification than his close friend Charlie accorded him.

In addition, Odrich, a trained dentist, appears in the Foundation files on Kelman in April 1965, close in time to when Kelman began to formally study the Cavitron for cataract surgery. Joan stated that Charlie knew of the Cavitron since 1962, before Charlie and Ron met, and Ron agreed with her on this point. Moreover, Ron has been consistent in every conversation with me that his major role was to urge caution regarding intraocular use of the Cavitron, rather than spurring Charlie on in this regard. Still, Norman Medow, who knew both Kelman and Odrich's sons during the early days of phacoemulsification, insists that the original epiphany that the Cavitron could be used for cataract surgery occurred at Odrich's office. Medow recalls that Kelman consistently indicated that he was at Odrich's office having a dental check-up when Kelman had the epiphany that the Cavitron could be used for eye surgery, travelled to the lab to get a crystalline lens for experimentation, and returned to Odrich's office to try the Cavitron on the lens.

It seems Charlie had a number of contacts from the dental world who could have provided information about the Cavitron—his wife, Kuhn, and Odrich—and the precise role each played and the timing may never be known with certainty. It is tempting to speculate on a scenario which would explain most of the known facts. Perhaps, Charlie was discouraged with the progress of his research reasonably early (1963 or 1964), when Ron Odrich did not have a Cavitron, but Larry Kuhn did. Charlie took a break from work, and visited the nearby office of his good friend Ron, for a dental checkup. Charlie and Ron looked at all the dental devices in the office, and discussed the likelihood that each of them could work on cataracts. One of the two friends (Charlie or Ron) brought up the idea of using the Cavitron for cataract surgery. Charlie could have known of the Cavitron from his wife, or from the January 1963 front page New York Times story, and Ron, of course, was intimately familiar with this tool, even though he was wary of the thermal damage it could produce in the mouth and in the eye. The two discussed how the thermal challenge could be mitigated, and Charlie left the office hastily. He got a cataract from his nearby laboratory (potentially a cataract sourced from the eye bank or from an animal) and drove out to Larry's office. Larry took Charlie to the hygiene room to show him the device, and Charlie was elated. Larry noticed that the Cavitron just seemed to push the cataract around without emulsifying it, but Charlie persuaded Larry that the technique needed more study. The two arranged to meet at Charlie's lab to test Larry's Cavitron on eyes under the microscope. There, Charlie could see that the Cavitron showed promise in emulsifying the lens. After working with Larry's Cavitron for some period of time in his lab, Kelman contacted the manufacturer in February 1965 to build a device with aspiration. When Kelman retold the tale in his autobiography, he had Larry stand in for the activity of both dentists for the sake of a good, simple story.

## Personal Follow-Up

Anton Banko left Cavitron and started surgical design in July 1968. He patented a system for pars plana vitrectomy in September 1968. In April 1986, Banko felt ill and had to be hospitalized. Within 4 weeks, he died of a severe autoimmune disease, at the age of 58 years.[122]

Charlie mentored Kuhn's son, Kerry, played the saxophone at Kerry's medical school graduation in 1973 and flew him in a helicopter from Long Island to New Jersey to watch eye surgeries.

Odrich's sons Marc and Steven became ophthalmologists. Before that time, Marc had worked as a teenager in Kelman's office in the summers of 1973 to 1975.

Charlie and Joan had three children and divorced in 1979. In 1989, Charlie married Ann and had three sons.

Charlie and Larry both retired to Florida in 1996. Charlie lived in Boca Raton, while Larry lived in Woodlands and Bocaire. Larry became known for sculpting in marble. The Kelman and Kuhn families continued to socialize after they moved to Florida. Larry's son, Kerry, visited Charlie and Ann, at their home there.

Charlie was diagnosed with lung cancer and passed away in 2004. Ron Odrich spoke at his memorial. That year, Charles Kelman was posthumously awarded the Lasker Award for medical science.

## Conclusions

Charles Kelman was probably the first in the United States to perform cryoextraction of cataracts and was the first anywhere to use for cataract extraction an advanced cryoprobe, which permitted the surgeon to apply and release cooling of the probe. Kelman was the first in the United States to publish experimental cryosurgery in animals for retinal detachments. This work helped to initiate a renaissance in this retinal technique, which had fallen by the wayside since its origination in Europe in the 1930s.

It was perhaps as early as 1962 when Charles Kelman learned of the Cavitron, an ultrasonic dental cleaning tool, from his fiancée, who worked in the dental office of Larry Kuhn. The fact that Charlie and Larry were together for multiple early, exploratory steps in phacoemulsification development suggests that this early phase was a collaborative effort between the two men. In addition, another dentist, Ronald Odrich, was a close friend of Kelman during the development of phacoemulsification.

---

122 Hawlina, 2013; Hawlina, 2014.

In fact, Odrich worked in Kelman's lab at the time, and likely made important contributions to the phacoemulsification project.

Kelman initially pursued other ideas for cataract surgery, including cryoextraction (by 1962) and chemical digestion (possibly in 1963). His first grant, which covered small incision cataract surgery, became active in January 1964. In the first year of the grant, he studied various mechanical means to macerate the lens. The first test of the Cavitron on the lens of a cat, conducted by Kelman with his dentist, Larry Kuhn, did not appear to be effective. Nonetheless, Kelman forged ahead. Beginning in February 1965, Kelman and Cavitron engineer Anton Banko began working on phacoemulsification. The first time the Cavitron was able to remove a cataract in any species in a manner deemed a success was in a cat's eye on March 23, 1966. The first two cataract phacoemulsifications in two human patients took place between April and June of 1967. Charles Kelman's pursuit of small incision cataract surgery began earlier and played out over a longer period of time than is generally recognized.

# References


Allen ED. Understanding Phacoemulsification. I. Principles of the Machinery. *Eur J Implant Ref Surg*. 1995;7:247-250.

American Medical Association. *Transactions of the Section on Ophthalmology of the American Medical Association at the 111th Annual Session*. 1962; 108.

Anker D. *Through My Eyes: the Charlie Kelman Story*. Production of WLIW New York; 2010. Available from: https://www.youtube.com/watch?v=IJoUlt9NIkk

Anonymous. Report on Meetings. *J Pediatr Ophthalmol Strabismus*. 1964 Jan 1;1(1):68-69.

Associated Press. Freezing technique in brain area cited. *Utica Observer-Dispatch*. Aug 30, 1961; 22.

Berens C, Sheppard LB. Clinical and experimental consideration of cycloelectrolysis and cyclodiathermy. *Am J Ophthalmol*. 1960 Oct 1;50(4):599-613.

Bietti G. Surgical intervention on the ciliary body: new trends for the relief of glaucoma. *J Am Med Assoc*. 1950 Mar 25;142(12):889-897.

Bourke-White M, Eisenstaedt A. A brave woman's own story. Miss Bourke-White's fight against crippling disease. *Life*. June 22, 1959; 101-108.

*Cavitron Corp. v. Ultrasonic Research Corporation*. United States District Court, Miami. No. 66-856-Civ. March 18, 1969. Available from: https://casetext.com/case/cavitron-corp-v-ultrasonic-research-corporation Accessed November 4, 2023.

Cooper IS. Cryogenic surgery of the basal ganglia. *JAMA*. Aug. 18, 1962; 600-604.

Cooper IS. *The Vital Probe: My Life as a Brain Surgeon*. New York: Norton; 1981.

Fields S. Invents Icy Sight Saver. *Daily News*. May 18, 1965.

Garrison FH, Stockman FJ. *Index Medicus: a Monthly Classified Record of the Current Medical Literature of the World*. Second Series. Washington, DC: Carnegie Institution; Jan-Dec 1918: 471.

Harris GS. Alpha-chymotrypsin in cataract surgery. *Can Med Assoc J*. 1961 Jul 7;85(4):186.

Hawlina M. Forgotten Giant. *Eurotimes*. December 10, 2013. Available from: https://escrs. org/eurotimes//forgotten-giant/

Hawlina M. Anton Banko (Presentation). Winter ESCRS meeting in Ljubljana in 2014.

Hickey J. Eye Surgery Improved. *Boston Sunday Advertiser*, Boston. Oct 11, 1964: 40.

Hughes WF. Gargantuan Academy. *Arch Ophthalmol*. 1962 Jan 1;67(1):3-4.

Irvine AR. The Lens and Vitreous. *Arch Ophthalmol*. 1962 Apr 1;67(4):511-527.

Jacobson JS. *The Greatest Good: A History of the John A. Hartford Foundation*. New York: The Foundation; 1984.

Kelman CD. Cryosurgery of retinal detachment and other ocular conditions. *Eye Ear Nose Throat Monthly*. January 1963;42:42-46.

Kelman CD. *Further Applications of Freezing Techniques to Eye Surgery. Manhattan Eye, Ear, and Throat Hospital*. John A. Hartford Foundation grant application. November 18, 1963. John A. Hartford Foundation.

Kelman CD, Cooper IS. Cryophthalmic surgery. A resume of the text presented with the film. Presented at the American Academy of Ophthalmology and Otolaryngology, Oct. 20-25, 1963, New York. *Trans Am Acad Ophthalmol Otolaryngol* 1964 Nov-Dec;68:1009-1011.

Kelman CD. *Atlas of Cryosurgical Techniques in Ophthalmology*. Saint Louis: Mosby; 1966.

Kelman CD. Phaco-emulsification and aspiration. A new technique of cataract removal. A preliminary report. *Am J Ophthalmol*. 1967;64(1):23-35.

Kelman CD. Cataract emulsification and aspiration. *Trans Ophthalmol Soc UK*. 1970 Jan 1;90:13-22.

Kelman CD. Symposium: Phacoemulsification. History of emulsification and aspiration of senile cataracts. Presented at the American Academy of Ophthalmology and Otolaryngology, Dallas, Sep. 16-20, 1973. *Trans Am Acad Ophthalmol Otolaryngol*. 1974 Jan-Feb;78(1):OP5-13.

Kelman CD. *Through My Eyes. The Story of a Surgeon who Dared to Take on the Medical World*. New York: Crown; 1985.

Kelman CD. Phaco-emulsification and aspiration: A progress report. *Am J Ophthalmol*. 1969 Apr 1;67(4):464-477.

Kelman CD. *Ridley Medal Lecture. Advances in Intraocular Lens Implant*. New Delhi: MacMillan India. March 26-29, 1990: 1-7.

Kelman CD. The history and development of phacoemulsification. *Int Ophthalmol Clin*. 1994 Apr 1;34(2):1-2.

Kelman CD. *Cryocataract surgery. The History of Modern Cataract Surgery*. The Hague, Netherlands: Kugler; 1998: 97-106.

Kelman CD. *History of phacoemulsification. The History of Modern Cataract Surgery*. The Hague, Netherlands: Kugler; 1998: 123-130.

Krwawicz T. Intracapsular extraction of intumescent cataract by application of low temperature. *Brit J Ophthalmol*. 1961;45:279.

Krwawicz T. Dalsze wyniki operacji zaćmy peczniejącej przy zastosowaniu krioekstraktora [Further results of surgery of intumescent cataracts with the use of cryo-extraction]. *Klinika Oczna* 1961;31:201-203.

Krwawicz T. Further experience with intracapsular cataract extraction by application of low temperature. *Br J Ophthalmol*. 1963 Jan;47(1):36.

Lincoff HA, McLean JM, Nano H. Cryosurgical treatment of retinal detachment. *Trans Am Acad Ophthalmol Otolaryngol*. 1964;68:412-432.

*Look Magazine*. July 17, 1962. Bing Crosby, March for Peace. Available from: magazines-byjoseph.com/product/look-magazine-july-17-1962/ Accessed Sep. 22, 2023.

Lowe E. Meet Dr. Everything. *Newsday*. Melville, NY; July 25, 1976: 7-10.

Maltz M. *Psycho-Cybernetics*. New York: Pocket; 1960.

Moskin JR, Karales JH. New attack on a dread disease: Urgent search for a cure. *Look*. July 17, 1962: 67-72. Retrieved from: https://magazinesbyjoseph.com/

Newell FW. The American Academy of Ophthalmology and Otolaryngology. *Am J Ophthalmol*. 1962 Dec 1;54(6):1153-1155.

Newell FW. Irving H. Leopold, MD. *Trans Am Ophthalmol Soc*. 1993;91:14.

No author listed. Brain Tissue Frozen in Surgical Technique. *Columbus Evening Dispatch*, Aug. 31, 1961: 53.

No author listed. A red-hot hundred. Gallery of young leaders of the big breakthrough. *Life*. Sep. 14, 1962: 4-19.

No author listed. Charles Kelman, MD: ophthalmologist, visionary, entertainer. *Ocular Surgery News*. New York: Helio; January 15, 2002.

No author listed. John A. Hartford Foundation records: C. Kelman, Grants, Series 3. Box 279. *Rockefeller Archives*. 1963-1972.

Odrich RB, Kelman CD. Cryotherapy, a new and experimental approach to the treatment of periodontal disease. *Periodontics*. 1967 Nov 1;5(6):313-317.

Rezaei KA, Abrams GW. The history of retinal detachment surgery. In: *Primary Retinal Detachment: Options for Repair*. Berlin, Heidelberg: Springer; 2005: 1-24.

Scheie HG, Frayer WC, Spencer RW. Cyclodiathermy: A clinical and tonographic evaluation. *AMA Arch Ophthalmol*. 1955;53(6):839-846.

Schoeler F. Experimentelle Erzeugung von Aderhaut-Netzhautentzündung durch Kohlensäure-schnee. Klin *Monatsbl Augenheilkd*. 1918;60(1):1.

Smothers R. Irving Cooper, man of science and arts. *New York Times*. Sep. 25, 1977;Section 22:1,4.

Vachon B. Cataract surgery: a different tune—can a saxophone player find happiness as an eye surgeon. *Saturday Review*. New York. April 15, 1972; 45-49.

Wilson JS. The jazz doctors' prescribe music as best therapy. *New York Times*. October 10, 1971;Section A:9.

Wilson JS. Jazz at Noon—Anyone Can Have Lunch With Jam. *New York Times*. May 25, 1975;Section 2:109.

Wudka E, Leopold IH. Experimental Studies of the Choroidal Vessels: V. Hemodynamic Observations. *AMA Arch Ophthalmol*. 1957 Nov 1;58(5):710-724.

# 3. The Phacoemulsification Era (1967)

**Theodore T. Wu, MD, PhD**

The advent of phacoemulsification in 1967 ushered in a new era of cataract surgery. Phacoemulsification (or "phaco," as it is often called) was a quantum leap forward at the time of its invention. The technique represented a major advance over extra- and intracapsular cataract extraction (ECCE and ICCE) in terms of safety and efficacy. Although its adoption was slow at first, by the late 1980s, phaco became the dominant technique for cataract removal in the United States, and by the 1990s, phaco was the dominant technique for cataract removal in the developed world. By 2021, over 4 million cataract surgeries per year are performed in the United States alone, and the majority of those cases are performed using phacoemulsification. Twenty-eight million cataract surgeries are performed each year worldwide.[1]

Phacoemulsification was developed by and first published in 1967 by Dr. Charles Kelman (Fig. 1). His work and perseverance are legendary. However, this new technique could not have succeeded without the help of many talented doctors who learned phaco and taught the technique to others. Some doctors were quick to adopt the new technique, but most were not.

Cataract surgery also benefited from the ingenuity of physicians and scientists who continued to improve the machines, instruments, and surgical techniques related to cataract surgery. In addition, the development of refractive surgery, photorefractive keratectomy (PRK) in 1987, and laser-assisted in situ keratomileusis (LASIK) in 1988 eventually led to US Food and Drug Administration (FDA) approval of femtosecond laser-assisted cataract surgery (FLACS) in 2010.[2]

Success in the operating room was only one hurdle. Because Dr. Kelman attended medical school in Europe, he had no strong ties with any senior "establishment" ophthalmologists in the United States.[3] This created a significant obstacle when he tried to introduce his new surgical technique to his colleagues. He had to overcome staunch resistance and skepticism from the existing ophthalmology establishment before his technique became widely accepted. Yet he persisted with his vision of a faster, safer, more effective cataract surgery method. Dr. Kelman even advocated for phaco on the Johnny Carson show and in front of an FDA panel, with the help of the famous TV doctor, Dr. Marcus Welby (Fig. 2).[4]

---

1 Lindstrom 2021.

2 Krueger 2013.

3 Kelman 1985.

4 Kelman 2006.

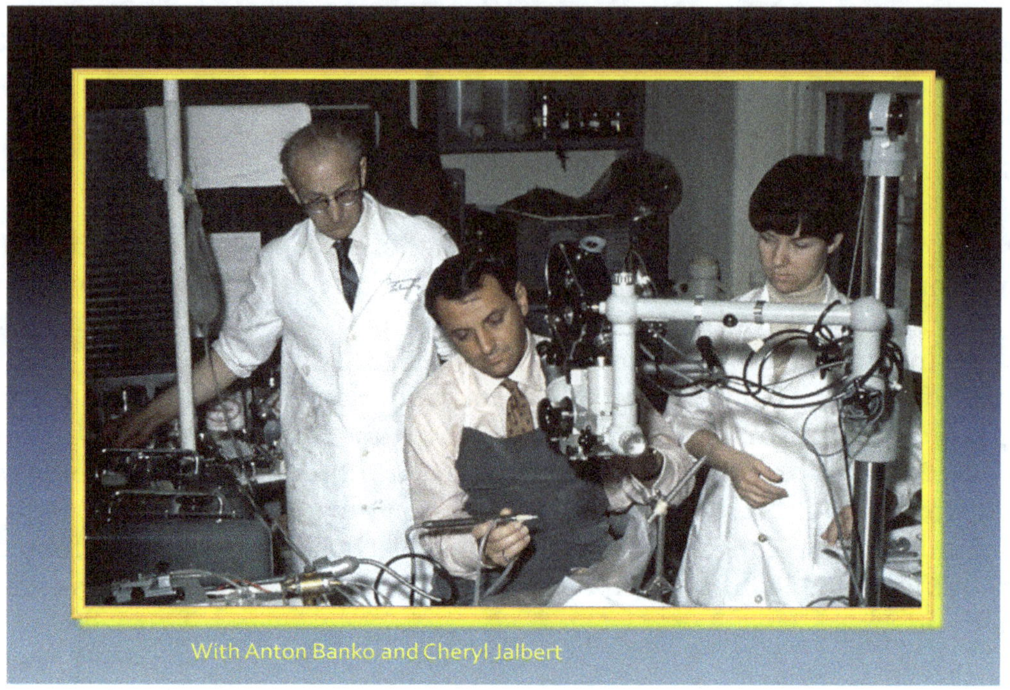


**Fig. 1.** Dr. Kelman and associates.

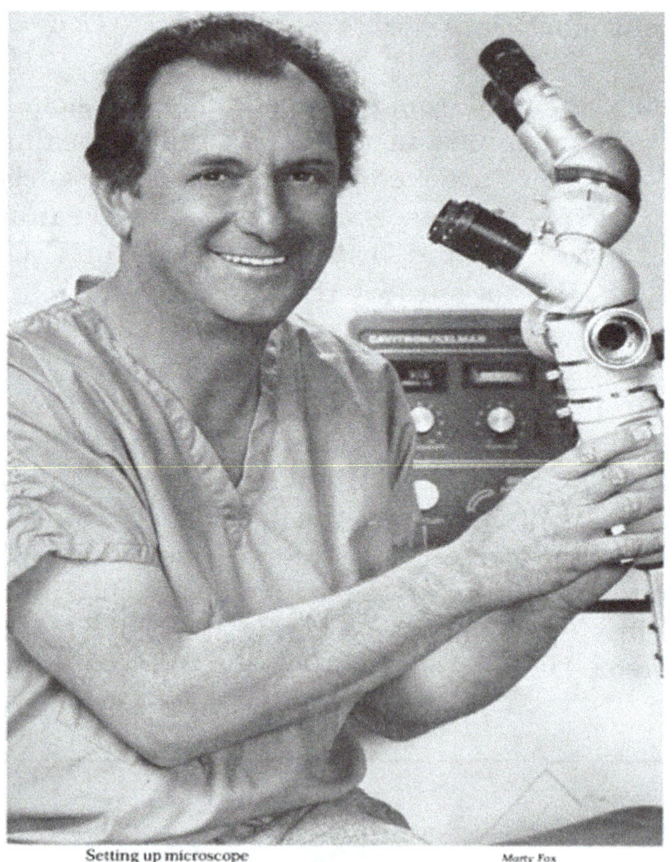


**Fig. 2.** Dr. Charles Kelman at the microscope.

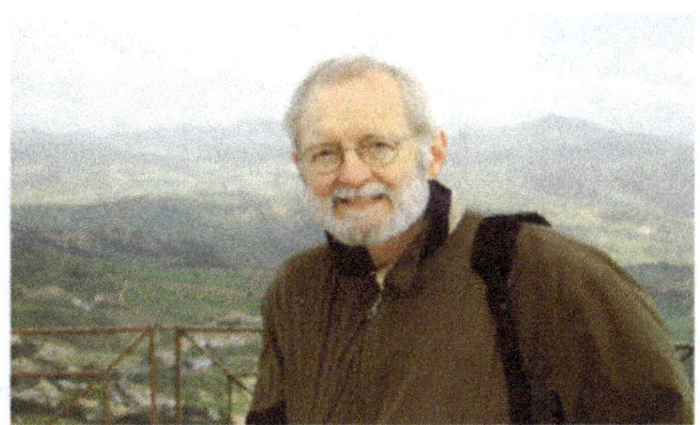

**Fig. 3.** Dr. Jared Emery.

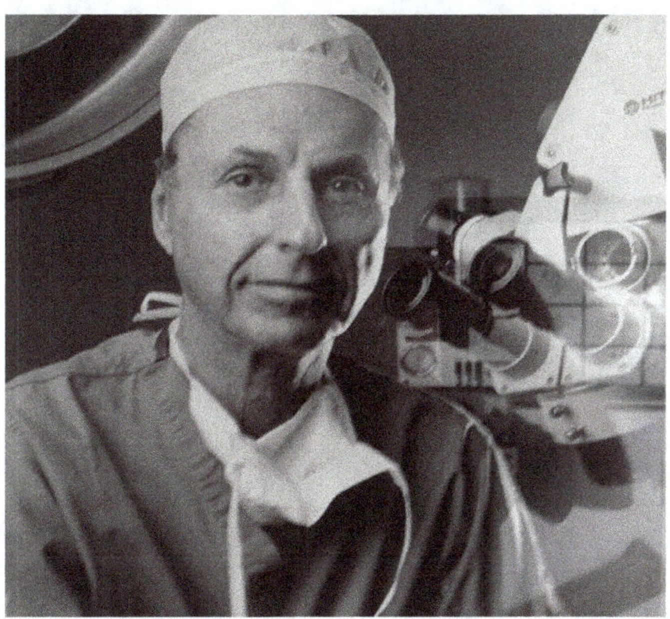

**Fig. 4.** Dr. Sinskey, early career.

Dr. Kelman taught phaco to two young doctors— Dr. Jared Emery and Dr. Robert Sinskey at the first phaco course taught in New York in 1972 (Figs. 3 and 4).

According to Dr. Douglas Koch:

Jared promptly went to the lab in evenings and weekends to validate its safety with numerous studies—and only after that did he offer it to patients. Then he did something that truly changed the landscape: he taught 3-day courses to train physicians, which included his performing live surgery broadcast to attendees over closed-circuit television…. In forty courses over eight years, he trained about 1,000, or nearly 10% of U.S. ophthalmologists. Jerry also traveled around the world teaching phaco and many other aspects of cataract surgery to international colleagues.[5]

---

5  Koch, D. Personal Communication, 2021 May 10.

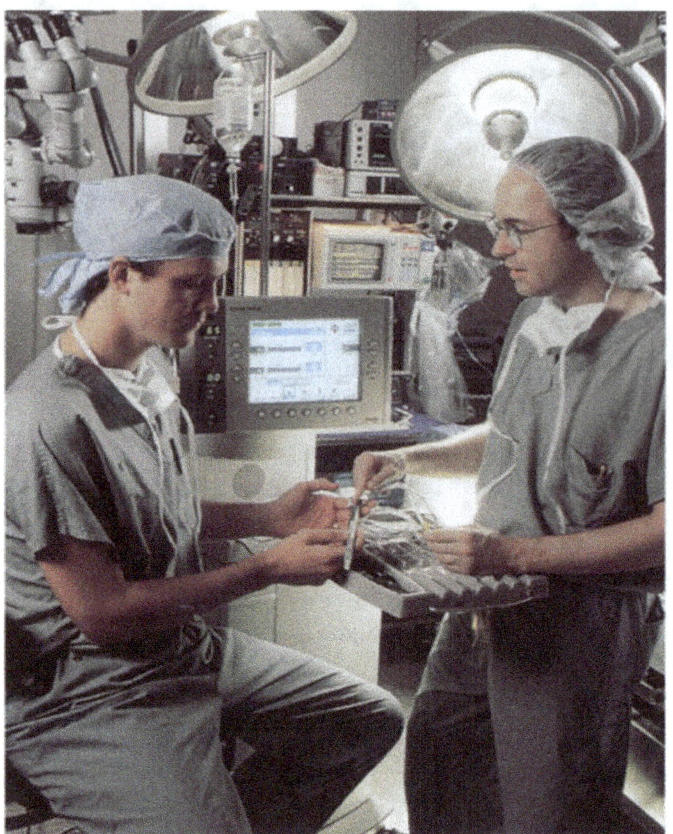

**Fig. 5.** Dr. Doug Koch with a resident.

One of Dr. Emery's residents at Baylor College of Medicine was Dr. Douglas Koch himself (in 1979) (Fig. 5).

According to Dr. Richard Packard, phaco was considered "ridiculous" or even grounds for malpractice in the early 1970s.[6] Mainstream ophthalmologists were still uneasy with phaco, as late as 1974. The nickname for phaco at the time was "buccaneer surgery":[7]

> …the American Academy of Ophthalmology (AAO) commissioned him [Dr. Emery] to conduct a study comparing traditional cataract surgery to phaco. Data that he collected demonstrated that phaco was as effective and safe as older techniques. He shared these data with the New York surgeon representing the AAO… and the surgeon told him that he wanted Jared to pull the paper. He faced intense pressure by this individual and others to suppress the results, but he staunchly resisted. His study was the critical step that brought phaco into the mainstream of ophthalmology and a turning point in transforming cataract surgery.[8]

---

6 Donnenfeld 2017.

7 Koch, D. Personal Communication, 2021 May 10.

8 Koch, D. Personal Communication, 2021 May 10.

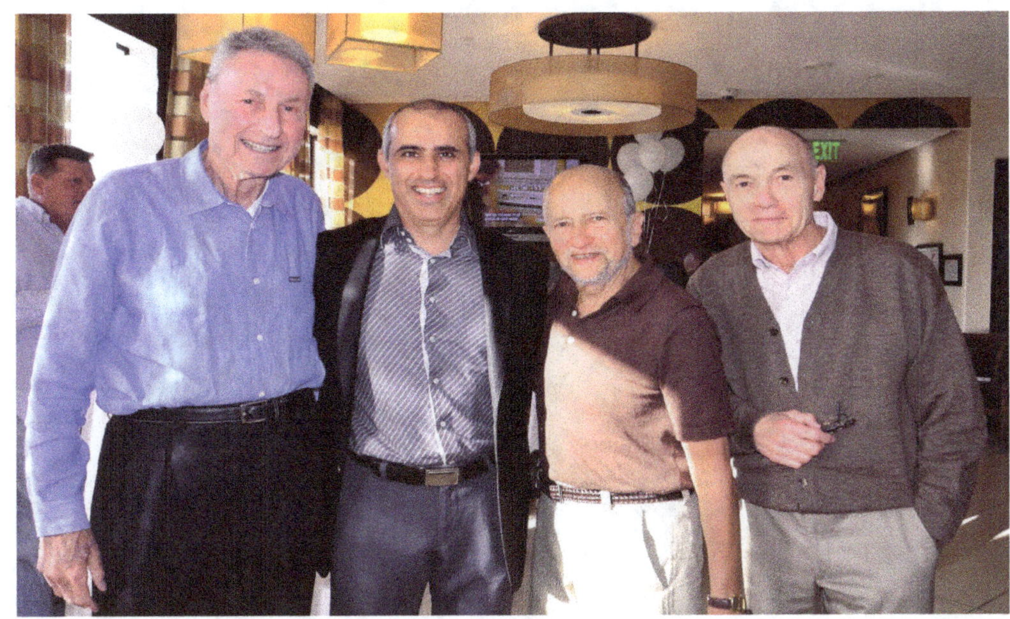

**Fig. 6.** Dr. Robert Sinskey and associates.

According to Dr. Richard Lindstrom, surgeons had a difficult time learning phaco technique and how to properly use an operating microscope.[9] In addition, the wound still needed to be opened to 6 mm to accommodate a nonfoldable intraocular lens (IOL), and early phaco cases caused significant corneal edema and iris damage.[10] Dr. Lindstrom estimates that no more than 100 surgeons in the United States were doing phaco in the early 1970s.[11]

In the mid-1970s, phaco became less popular while the surgical establishment stuck with intracapsular cataract surgery and the popular Binkhorst and Choyce lenses. According to Dr. Robert Sinskey (Fig. 6):

> I introduced phacoemulsification to surgeons in Rio de Janeiro, Brazil and to surgeons in more than 41 countries during the next 15 to 20 years. Resistance within the profession to phacoemulsification was strong, particularly in Europe, not only because of the difficult learning curve, but because of the procedure's cost.[12]

Early Cavitron machines cost about $40,000 (Fig. 7).[13]

---

9 Donnenfeld 2017.

10 Donnenfeld 2017.

11 Donnenfeld 2017.

12 Sinskey 2006.

13 Mitchell 2006.

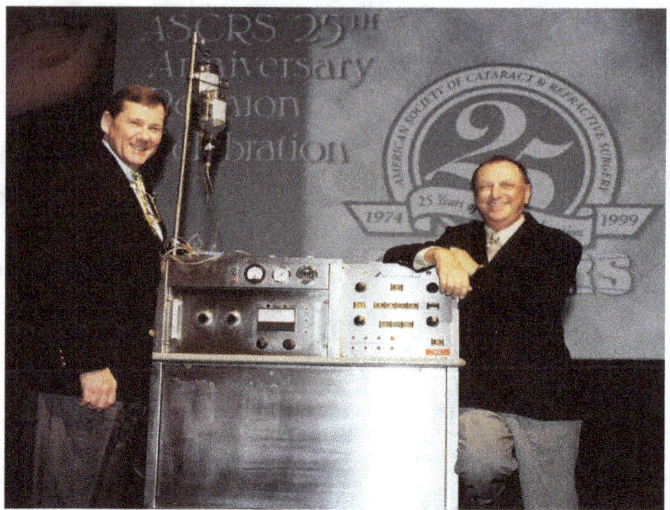

**Fig. 7.** Henry Mitchell with Charles Kelman and a Cavitron machine.

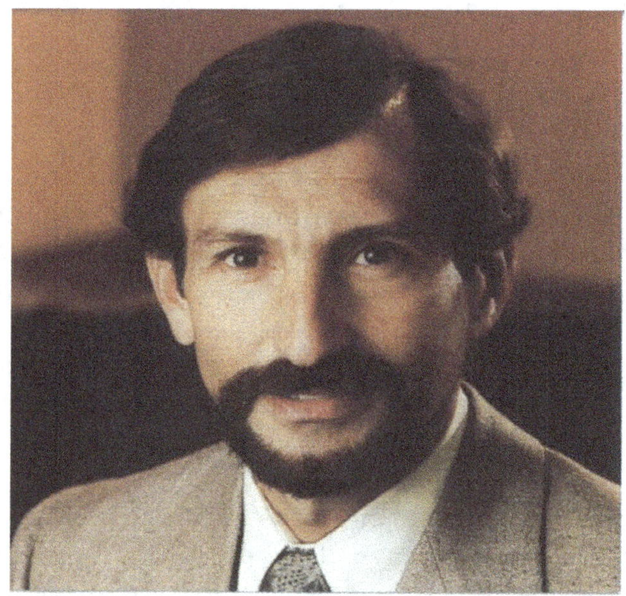

**Fig. 8.** Richard Mackool.

Dr. Richard Mackool was trained at the Manhattan Eye and Ear Infirmary in the early 1970s. Initially, he practiced cataract surgery on animal eyes in Dr. Kelman's laboratory. He describes his first phaco experience as "very tense" (Fig. 8).[14]

The (first) Cavitron instrument was primitive by today's standards. The maximum vacuum that could be used was 50 mm Hg, and the anterior chamber was unstable. Near the end of the case, a tear in the posterior capsule occurred, but fortunately the cataract was not dense and I was able to remove the entire nucleus and cortex. In

14  Mackool, Richard. Personal Communication, 2022 March 6.

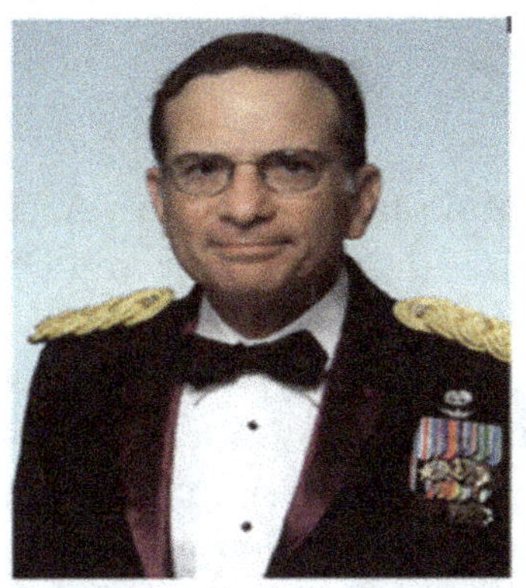


**Fig. 9A.** Dr. Hal Kushner.

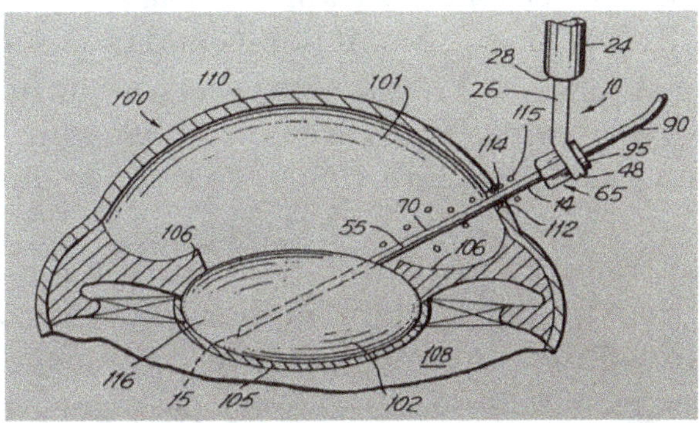

**Fig. 9B.** Patent by John P. Shock filed in 1972 for ultrasonic cataract removal apparatus.

the early-mid 1970's we were not yet using intraocular lenses, had no viscoelastics, phaco was done either in the anterior chamber (Kelman technique) or iris plane (Kratz technique), and vitrectomy was done with sponges and scissors.[15]

Dr. Hal Kushner is a former Army Flight Surgeon who spent 65 months as a prisoners of war (POW) during the Vietnam War (Fig. 9A). After the war, he did his residency in ophthalmology from 1974 to 1977 in the Army at Brooke Army Medical Center in San Antonio, Texas. His Chief of Ophthalmology was Dr. John Shock, who invented and developed an instrument called the "J Shock Phacofragmenter"—an ultrasonic handpiece without any sophisticated fluidics (just an IV line) (Fig. 9B). In residency, Dr. Kushner did a few cataracts using the Shock Phacofragmenter and several planned ECCE, but the majority of cases were done using ICCE. (The Shock Phacofragmenter was used for many years by retinal surgeons for nuclear fragmentation but was never marketed as a cataract device.)

---

15 Mackool, Richard. Personal Communication, 2022 March 6.

Dr. Kushner recounted:

> In 1981, I attended an ECCE and phaco course in Atlanta given by Cavitron/Cooper Vision. The course was taught by Dr Jess Lester and Dr Barry Thrasher, both Atlanta ophthalmologists, and utilized the Cooper Vision Cavitron machine. I met Henry Mitchell at that course which also had Dr Bob Loftus (a PhD in Anthropology who taught phaco!). In 1983, I started doing phaco and I went down to Miami to watch Dr. Clayman and Dr. Jaffe operate, and then later up to Calgary, Canada to spend a day watching Dr. Howard Gimbel's masterful surgery. Henry Mitchell came to Daytona about this time and trained me on the phaco machine… He taught me, as no one in my town was doing phaco then. I started with softer cataract lenses, widely dilated pupils (this is before viscoelastic) and 'easy' cases. Although I had used the microscope since my second year in residency, I didn't appreciate the nuances and subtleties of the posterior capsule until Henry Mitchell put an observer tube on my hospital microscope and scrubbed with me. It was a revelation…. I didn't start doing 'hard cases' until 1987 or so… small pupils and hard lenses; but what really revolutionized my and others' practice patterns was the capsulorhexis as described by (Dr.) Gimbel and the foldable lenses which I think were popularized by Tom Mazzocco on the West Coast in the late 1980s. That made phaco really popular.[16]

The Mazzocco IOL was introduced in 1984. It was the first foldable silicone plate IOL. This IOL could be introduced through a 3-mm incision—the "Mazzocco Taco."[17] Combined with innovations in phaco equipment and better techniques, the advantages of phaco over ECCE and ICCE became much clearer— lower postoperative astigmatism, clearer corneas, and a lower rate of retinal detachment. By 1985, 50% of cataract surgeries were performed by phaco, and by 2000, 90% of US surgeons were performing phaco.[18]

## Development of the Coaxial Microscope

Modern microsurgery would not be possible without the development of the ophthalmic surgical microscope. Excellent summaries of the development of the surgical microscope have been presented.[19] A timeline of important developments in the history of the ophthalmic surgical microscope are presented in Table 1.

Even though the ophthalmic surgical microscope was available for use in 1966, adoption of the microscope for routine eye procedures was somewhat slow at first. According to Dr. Ramon Castroviejo in 1967,

---

16  Kushner H. Personal Communication, 2022 February.

17  Sinskey 2006.

18  Minassian, Rosen, Dart, et al. 2001.

19  Keeler 2020, Ma 2021.

**Table 1.** Timeline of important developments in the history of the ophthalmic surgical microscope

| Year | Ophthalmic Surgical Microscope Development |
|---|---|
| 1938 | Otto Barkan performs intraocular surgery (goniotomy) under the microscope and uses the term "microsurgery." |
| 1946 | Richard Perritt uses a Bausch and Lomb microscope for ophthalmic surgical procedures. |
| 1948 | Hans Littmann develops a Zeiss microscope with coaxial illumination. |
| 1952 | Heinrich Harms modifies a Zeiss microscope by adding convergent eyepieces and an articulated arm attached to a solid moveable stand. |
| 1953 | OPMI® 1, the first surgical microscope, is developed in cooperation with leading surgeons Horst Wullstein (ENT) and Heinrich Harms (ophthalmology). |
| 1956 | Henri Dekking adds a support stand that allows foot control of lateral and transverse microscope movement and a knee lever to adjust focus. |
| 1956 | Jose Barraquer adds fine focusing via microscope footswitch. |
| 1961 | Hans Littmann develops the teaching microscope (Diploscope). |
| 1961 | Helmut Dannheim introduces improved foot pedal controls. |
| 1962 | Charles Keeler introduces the first motorized zoom microscope for surgical use. |
| 1965 | Zeiss OPMI II microscope is introduced with zoom optics from 2.5x to 53.5x. |
| 1966 | Zeiss OPMI 3 microscope is introduced specifically for ocular surgery. |
| 1970 | Zeiss microscope with 5x zoom system with continuous magnification adjustment is introduced. |
| 1984 | Wide-angle optics for Zeiss OPMI is introduced. |
| 1985 | Voice control system for Zeiss OPMI appears. |
| 2009 | Zeiss Lumera 700 is introduced for better visualization of lens and vitreous. |

Use of the microscope is a matter of personal adaptation. It requires patience as time is lost manipulating the instrument. Many people prefer to use loupe glasses which are made as strong as 5x now with a strong illuminating source of light. I use a microscope in all cases of corneal grafting, not during the whole operation, mainly for inserting stitches. I find that if the microscope is small enough, I can work as fast using it as without one, and with much more ease.[20]

---

20  Keeler 2020.

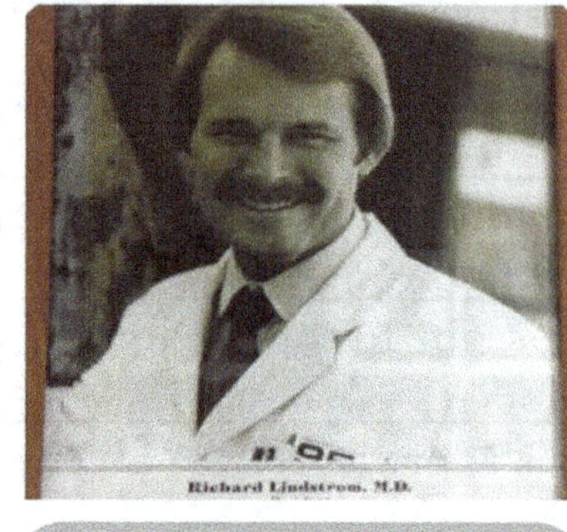



**Richard L. Lindstrom, MD:1978 Internal Medicine Internship, Ophthalmology Residency, then Three Fellowships: Minnesota, Texas and Utah.**

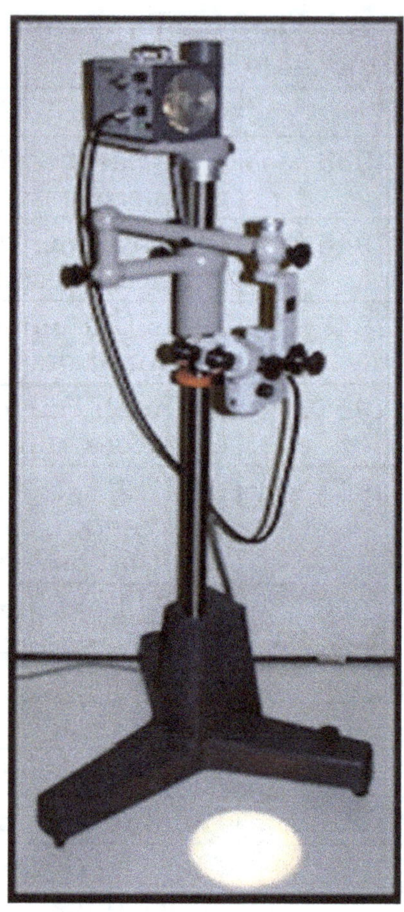

**Fig. 10.**  Early OPMI [Operations Mikroskop] Microscope.

Dr. Richard Lindstrom first used an operating microscope in the early 1970s (Figs. 10 and 11):

> Our Chairman, John Harris MD PHD was a member of the Ocular Microsurgery Study Group and adopted the Operating Microscope early for cataract and cornea. Zeiss OPMI [Operations Mikroskop] as I recall. First generation Zeiss, in any regard. It did have foot control for magnification and focus. But all [surgeries were] ICCE. Our Pediatric Ophthalmologist used Loupes.[21]

Around 1972, Dr. Richard Mackool began his training in ophthalmic microsurgery,

> I did about 150 Cataracts as a resident. The first 75 or so were done with loupes, and the last 75 with a microscope made by Weck. There was no coaxial illumination.[22]

---

21  Lindstrom, Richard. Personal Communication, March 2022.
22  Mackool, Richard. Personal Communication, 2022 March 6.

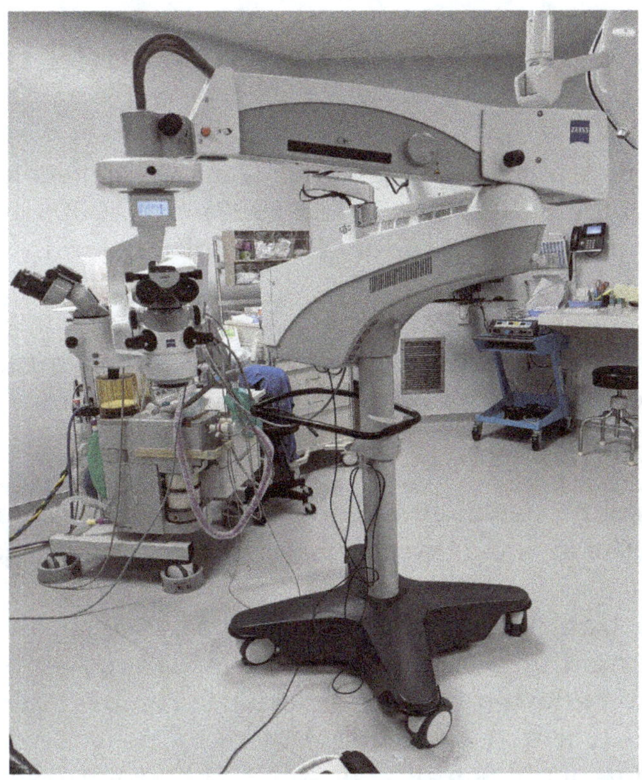

**Fig. 11.** Modern Zeiss OPMI [Operations Mikroskop] Lumera 700 Microscope.

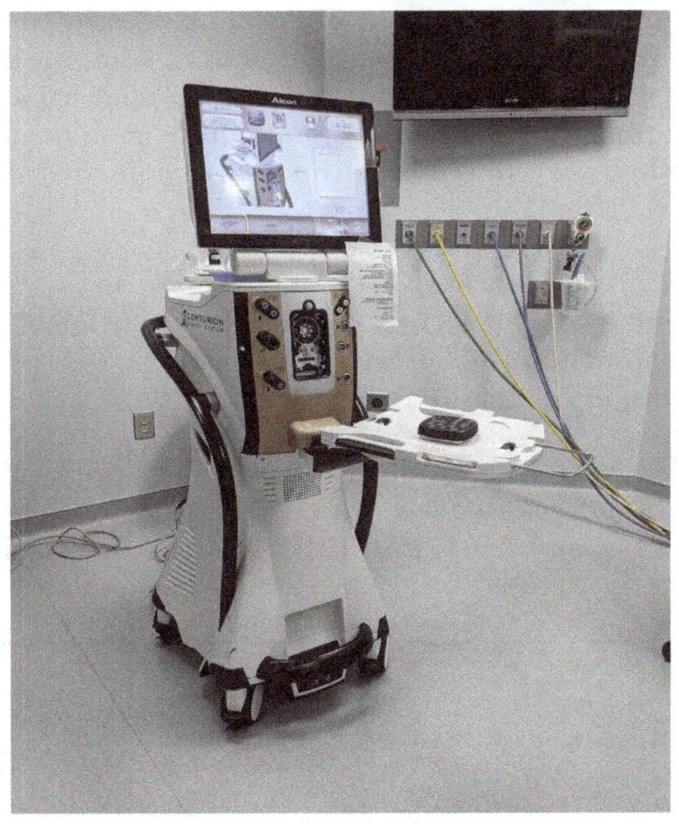

**Fig. 12.** Alcon Centurion Machine, introduced in 2013.

## Further Developments and Refinements in Cataract Surgery

Two other key developments that allowed phaco surgery to become widely successful were the development of foldable IOLs in the 1980s and 1990s and the development of viscoelastics, starting with the product launch of Healon in 1980, to protect the cornea during cataract surgery.

Better fluidics and wound construction also helped to maintain a stable anterior chamber during surgery, thereby improving surgical outcomes and protecting the corneal endothelium (Fig. 12).

Improved surgical techniques included development of the continuous curvilinear capsulorhexis in 1985, the divide-and-conquer method,[23] and phaco chop (D. Chang).[24]

In 2006, the introduction of bimanual phaco, performed through two 1.5 mm incisions, separated the irrigation and phaco/aspiration components so that each probe acted unopposed.[25] This allowed for less traumatic removal of cataracts in riskier patients—small pupils, corneal endothelial disease, pseudoexfoliation, traumatic cataracts, high myopia/elastic zonules, posterior polar cataracts, and a history of pars plana vitrectomy.[26] Perhaps of equal importance, a smaller incision resulted in less surgically induced astigmatism (SIA) at the wound site. Around the same time, microcoaxial phaco with torsional ultrasound was introduced. Microcoaxial phaco had the advantage of a faster learning curve compared to bimanual technique, about 60% more infusion than the typical 20-gauge irrigating chopper, better thermoprotection to prevent wound burns, and an incision large enough (2.0 to 2.2 mm) to implant a full-sized, 6-mm IOL without enlargement.[27] Both techniques are astigmatically neutral (Fig. 13).

The availability of intraoperative aberrometry, such as the Optiwave Refractive Analysis (ORA) system in 2011 (Alcon), aided in the correction of astigmatism during live surgery. This system allowed for fine-tuning of toric IOL placement within the eye and improved astigmatism management.[28]

In 2010, the LenSx system became the first FDA-approved FLACS (Fig. 14). The arrival of FLACS represented a confluence of traditional cataract surgery and refractive surgery, such as LASIK and PRK. For the first time, the Femto laser could be used for multiple steps of the cataract surgery, including (1) primary and

---

23  Ernest 2002.

24  Steinert 2009.

25  Rose 2006.

26  Rose 2006.

27  Osher 2008.

28  Fram, Masket, Wang 2015.

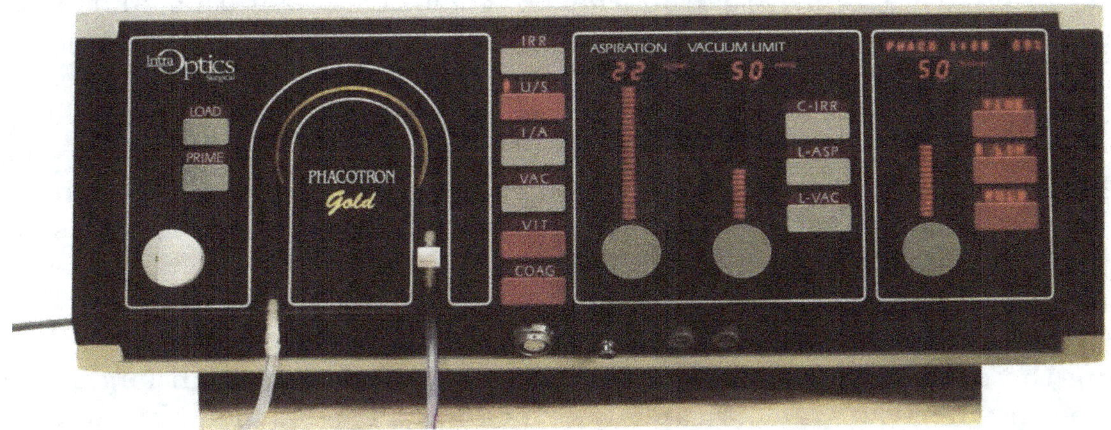

Dear Bob:

Thank you for responding to my request for an edited video of your surgical technique and accompanying commentary.

Your contribution regarding the technique of Slow Motion Phaco is highly important to phacoemulsification and I look forward to showing the videotape and crediting you for your achievement in this area.

With my thanks again and best wishes, I am

Sincerely yours,

Charles D. Kelman, M.D.

**Fig. 13.** Letter from Dr. Kelman to Dr. Osher.

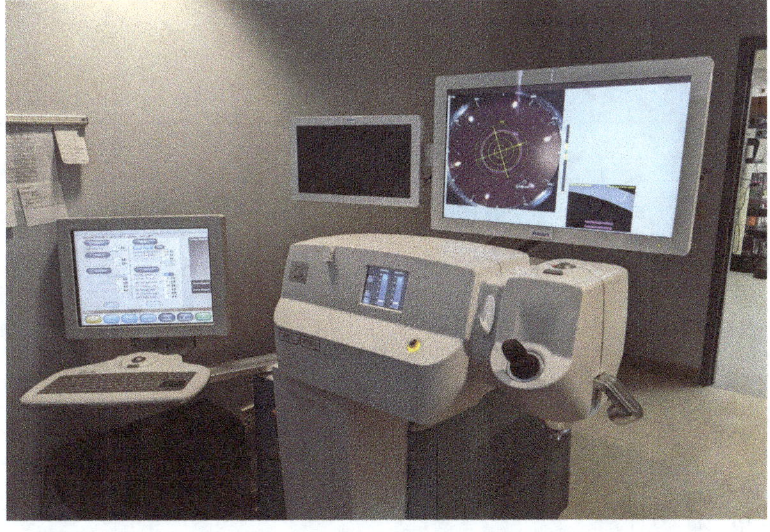

**Fig. 14.** LenSx Machine for femtosecond laser-assisted cataract surgery.

secondary wound creation, (2) capsulorhexis, (3) lens fragmentation, and (4) astigmatic correction via laser relaxing incisions. The Femto laser, by prechopping the nucleus, resulted in reduced phaco energy for each surgery (about 50% less) and reduced phaco time per case.[29] This was especially important in more challenging cases, such as Fuch's endothelial corneal dystrophy or high hyperopes with shorter axial length. FLACS also proved to be quite useful in pseudoexfoliation cases, because the prechopped nucleus was easier to remove and imparted less stress on the zonules during surgery.[30] In addition, FLACS was extremely useful for breaking up dense "Coca Cola" cataracts to reduce overall phaco energy. FLACS was also successful in performing a capsulorhexis in white cataracts, thereby avoiding the dreaded "Argentinian flag sign."[31] (The Argentinian flag sign was said to occur when the anterior capsule, which had been stained blue, split open in an uncontrolled fashion, exposing the white cataract.) FLACS can also be used in traumatic cataract cases involving damaged zonules.[32] I (TW) have observed that FLACS can be used for posterior polar cataracts, as customized treatment can be designed to avoid the weakest part of the capsule.

The ability to perfectly center and size the rhexis improved the effective lens position of the IOL, thus improving the predictability of the final refractive result.[33]

The biggest barrier to widespread adoption of FLACS was the cost of the equipment and cost to the patient. Another significant barrier was the learning curve for new FLACS surgeons.[34]

Several randomized controlled trials suggest that surgical outcomes are similar when comparing FLACS and conventional phaco surgery.[35] However, other studies suggest that FLACS may be beneficial in certain patient subgroups, such as white cataracts,[36] traumatic cataracts,[37] dense cataracts, corneal endothelial dystrophy,[38] and multifocal or extended depth-of-focus (EDOF) IOL implantation.[39] Also, eyes treated with FLACS may have faster visual recovery and earlier stabilization of refraction compared to conventional phaco.[40]

---

29 Assaf 2021.

30 Krueger 2013, p. 182.

31 Zhu 2019.

32 Huang 2020.

33 Krueger 2013.

34 Christy 2017.

35 Roberts 2019; Schweitzer 2020.

36 Zhu 2019.

37 Nagy 2012.

38 Al-Mohtaseb 2017.

39 Lee, Song, Kim et al. 2019.

40 Conrad 2015.

Of concern is data that suggest that FLACS may be more proinflammatory than conventional phaco, leading to higher rates of postoperative corneal edema, early posterior capsular opacification, uveitis, and uncontrolled IOP.[41] Also, this proinflammatory effect may explain a trend toward greater frequency of cystoid macular edema in FLACS versus conventional phaco.[42] However, in over 1000 FLACS cases, I have not observed a higher rate of these complications when compared to phaco—perhaps the complication rate may depend on the particular surgeon, level of surgeon experience with FLACS, or the particular FLACS platform being used. (There are at least four FLACS platforms in commercial use in 2022.) Hopefully, the next generation of femtosecond laser technology will be less likely to induce inflammation during surgery and have fewer postoperative complications.

## Cataract Surgery: Future Directions...

What will the future hold for cataract surgery? Improved preoperative diagnostics will hopefully allow the surgeon to achieve the desired target refraction greater than 95% of the time. Better microscopes with integrated real-time diagnostics will allow better visualization of the cataract and allow for adjustments of IOL power and axis prior to IOL implantation. An integrated Femto/phaco machine will become the norm as FLACS becomes the predominant cataract surgery method over the next 25 years. Better Femto lasers with a gentler patient interface, higher resolution optical coherence tomography (OCT), and less induced inflammation will improve patient comfort and outcomes. Furthermore, the next generation of intraocular implants will allow patients to see close up, intermediate distance, and far with adjustable manifest refraction and adjustable light transmission. Finally, what role will artificial intelligence and robots play in cataract surgery planning and actual surgery? Perhaps one day the surgeon will perform multiple surgeries at the same time from a single control room at a remote location.

## References


Al-Mohtaseb Z, He X, Yesilirmak N, et al. Comparison of corneal endothelial cell loss between two femtosecond laser platforms and standard phacoemulsification. *J Refract Surg.* 2017 Oct 1;33(10):708-712.

Assaf AH, Aly MG, Zaki RG, et al. Femtosecond laser-assisted cataract surgery in soft and hard nuclear cataracts: a comparison of effective phacoemulsification time. *Clin Ophthalmol.* 2021;15:1095-1099.

Christy JS, Nath M, Mouttapa F, et al. Learning curve of femtosecond laser-assisted cataract surgery: experience of surgeons new to femtosecond laser platform. *Indian J Ophthalmol.* 2017;65:683-689.

Conrad-Hengerer I, Al Sheikh M, Hengerer FH, et al. Comparison of visual recovery and refractive stability between femtosecond laser-assisted cataract surgery and standard phacoemulsification: six month follow-up. *J Cataract Refract Surg.* 2015 Jul;41(7):1356-1364.

Donnenfeld E. Phaco Turns 50. *EyeWorld* 2017 April:130-138.


---

41 Manning, Barry, Henry, et al. 2016.

42 Ewe 2015.

Ernest P. *Divide and Conquer Technique*. CRST; 2002 September.

Ewe S, Oakley CL, Abell RG, et al. Cystoid macular edema after femtosecond laser-assisted versus phacoemulsification cataract surgery. *JCRS*. 2015 Nov;41(11):2373-2378.

Fram NR, Masket S, Wang L. Comparison of intraoperative aberrometry, OCT-based IOL formula, Haigis-L, and Masket formulae for IOL power calculation after laser vision correction. *Ophthalmology*. 2015 Jun 1;122(6):1096-1101.

Huang PW, Huang WH, Tai YC, et al. Femtosecond laser-assisted cataract surgery in a patient with traumatic cataract and corneal opacity after LASIK: a case report. *BMC Ophthalmol*. 2020;20:218.

Keeler R. The history of the surgical microscope in ophthalmology. In: Leffler CT, ed. *The History of Glaucoma*. Amsterdam: Kugler, Wayenborgh; 2020:481-512.

Kelman C. *Through My Eyes*. New York, NY: Crown Publishers; 1985.

Kelman C. *The Genesis of Phacoemulsification*. Wayne, PA: CRST Europe; Sept 2006 (written 2004).

Krueger RR, Talamo, JH, Lindstrom RL. *Textbook of Refractive Laser Assisted Cataract Surgery (ReLACS)*. New York, NY: Springer; 2013.

Lee JA, Song WK, Kim JY, et al. Femtosecond laser-assisted cataract surgery versus conventional phacoemulsification: refractive and aberrometric outcomes with a diffractive multifocal intraocular lens. *J Cataract Refract Surg*. 2019 Jan;45(1):21-27.

Lindstrom R. Future of cataract surgery seems promising. *Ocul Surg News*, Feb 10, 2021:1-2.

Ma L, Fei B. Comprehensive review of surgical microscopes: technology development and medical applications. *J Biomed Opt*. 2021 Jan;26(1):010901.

Manning S, Barry P, Henry Y, et al. Femtosecond laser-assisted cataract surgery versus standard phacoemulsification cataract surgery: study from the European registry of quality outcomes for cataract and refractive surgery. *J Cataract Refract Surg*. 2016;42:1779-1790.

Minassian DC, Rosen P, Dart JKG, et al. Extracapsular cataract extraction compared with small incision cataract surgery by phacoemulsification: a randomised trial. *Br J Ophthalmol*. 2001;85:822-829.

Mitchell H. *The First Phaco Machines*. Wayne, PA: Bryn Mawr Communications; September 2006.

Nagy ZZ, Kranitz K, Takacs A, et al. Intraocular femtosecond laser use in traumatic cataracts following penetrating and blunt trauma. *J Refract Surg*. 2012 Feb;28(2):151-153.

Osher R. Micro-coaxial phaco, torsional ultrasound a perfect marriage, doctor says. *Ophthal Times*. 2008:1-2.

Roberts HW, Wagh VK, Sullivan DL, et al. A randomized controlled trial comparing femtosecond laser-assisted cataract surgery versus conventional phacoemulsification surgery. *J Cataract Refract Surg*. 2019 Jan;45(1):11-20.

Rose AD. *Bimanual Versus Coaxial*. Wayne, PA: Bryn Mawr Communications; 2006:1-13.

Schweitzer C, Brezin A, Cochener B, et al. Femtosecond Laser-assisted Versus Phacoemulsification Cataract Surgery (FEMCAT): a multicentre participant-masked randomised superiority and cost-effectiveness trial. *Lancet*. 2020 Jan 18;395(10219):212-224.

Sinskey R. *Phacoemulsification and IOLs*. Wayne, PA: Bryn Mawr Communications; September 2006.

Steinert R. *Cataract Surgery*. 3rd ed. New York, NY: Elsevier; 2009.

Zhu Y, Chen X, Xu W, et al. Lens capsule-related complications of femtosecond laser-assisted capsulotomy versus manual capsulotomy for white cataracts. *J Cataract Refract Surg*. 2019;45:337-342.

# A *New History of Cataract Surgery* consists of:



* Chapters origination from: *The History of Ophthalmology – The Monographs 15: The History of Glaucoma*